Current Cancer Research 2006

Deutsches Krebsforschungszentrum

German Cancer Research Center
in the Helmholtz Association

The Research Programs

Account for donations
Deutsche Bank Heidelberg
Bank code number
672 700 03
Account number
0157008

Greeting by the President of the Helmholtz Association

"Current Cancer Research" – Fascinating Insights into the German Cancer Research Center

The Helmholtz Association has an ambitious mission: leading edge research that contributes to solving the great and pressing challenges facing science, society and industry. With our 24 000 staff in 15 member research centers, an annual budget of more than two billion euros and program-based strategic orientation of our research, we are well equipped to fulfill this task. Our scientists work in six core fields: energy, earth and environment, health, key technologies, structure of matter, transport and space. It is our aim to answer fundamental questions in these ma-

jor areas. In practical terms, this means that our research aims to achieve relevant advances of knowledge, secure and enhance quality of life and create new practical solutions through knowledge transfer.

One example is our cancer research. Each year, over 200 000 people in Germany still die of cancer. To gain a better understanding of cancer causing mechanisms, identify risk factors, improve prevention, diagnose cancer earlier and more accurately and to find new treatment approaches – these are among the biggest challenges of medicine. To meet those, six research centers have joined competences and resources within our Program

"Cancer Research". Scientists of different disciplines such as molecular biologists, immunologists, physicists and doctors are working together to obtain relevant findings and enhance transfer of their results into clinical application.

The flagship of cancer research within the Helmholtz Association is the German Cancer Research Center (Deutsches Krebsforschungszentrum, DKFZ), which is recognized in Germany and other countries as a leading institute in this field. "Current Cancer Research" bears witness to the impressive performance of the Center, its comprehensive approach and broad range of methods. The work of the Center is currently

Prof. Dr. Jürgen Mlynek
President of the Helmholtz
Association

focused on six multidisciplin-
ary Research Programs: Cell
Biology and Tumor Biology,
Structural and Functional Genomics, Cancer Risk Factors and
Prevention, Tumor Immunology, Innovative Diagnostics
and Therapy, Infection and
Cancer. Readers will learn
about what is concealed behind
these as well as about the Center's commitment to general
tasks such as technology transfer and support of young researchers. In short, if you want
to know: What is leading edge
cancer research today? – then
this is a must-read book. May
it have many curious readers.

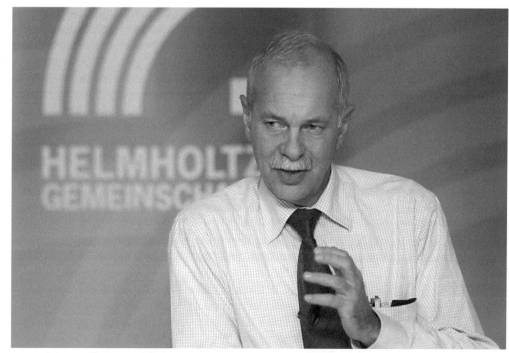

Research for the Sake of the Patients

In September 2005, an article published in the journal *Deutsches Ärzteblatt* attracted a great deal of attention. Under the heading "The underestimated advances in oncology", Professor Hermann Brenner reported on the long-term survival rates of cancer patients in Germany. Brenner, who now leads the Division of Clinical Epidemiology and Aging Research at the Deutsches Krebsforschungszentrum (German Cancer Research Center, DKFZ), had good news: Using a refined method of data analysis, he was able to prove that patients diagnosed with many of the common cancers today survive their diagnosis significantly longer than previously calculated. The most plausible expla-

nation for this is that tumors are detected earlier and treated better today than only a few years ago, or, in short, that the scientific efforts of the past few decades have resulted in visible, albeit small, advances.

To me, to every other staff member of the German Cancer Research Center, and also to doctors and scientists working in oncology throughout the world, these results are an encouraging signal: They show that our work is going in the right direction. It goes without saying that this is not a reason to become idle, but an incentive to further intensify our efforts in the future.

Far too many cancer patients still die of their disease. Although many breakthroughs have been achieved over the past decade at the levels of molecular and cell biology or genome research in terms of our understanding of the malignant transformation of cells, therapeutic advances – particularly in the treatment of several important cancers – have unfortunately been lagging behind substantially. At the same time, the results obtained in basic research often open up new avenues that lead us to specific, innovative treatment approaches. Now it is key to test these new approaches in close cooperation between research and clinical practice so that they can be applied for

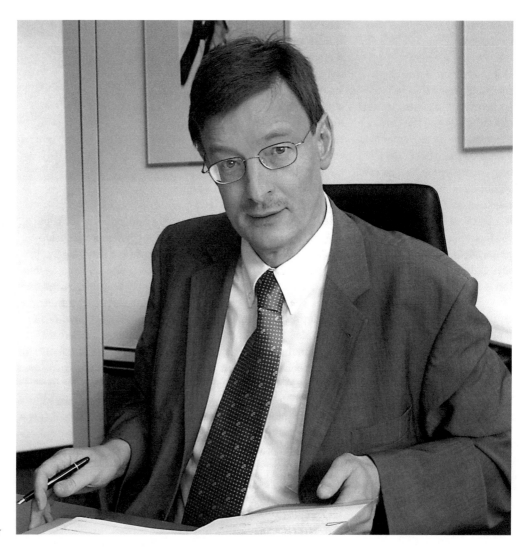

Prof. Dr. Otmar D. Wiestler,
Chairman and Scientific Director
of the German Cancer Research Center

the benefit of patients as soon as possible.

This was one of the chief reasons why we established, jointly with Heidelberg University Hospitals and the Thorax Clinic, the National Center for Tumor Diseases (NCT) Heidelberg in Summer 2003. The joint organization, which is portrayed in an article on page 152, is a platform that enables the collaborating partners to test promising developments from the Heidelberg research laboratories in clinical trials.

Usually it takes many years for a promising result in cancer research to make its way into clinical practice. A success story from our Center provides a good example: Back in the late 1980s, Harald zur Hausen and Lutz Gissmann had the crucial idea how to efficiently arm the immune system against cancer causing papillomaviruses. Today, almost two decades later, two pharmaceutical companies are releasing vaccines based on

these developments to protect women against cervical cancer. A great deal of work lies between an idea and a market launch: Extensive tests are needed to make sure that a new substance does not harm the body; the chemical structure of novel drugs needs to be optimized in a laborious process. All this lies beyond the possibilities of a research institute. This is why we intend to support our scientists in their work by providing a research and development platform for translational oncology in the future. The platform is intended to conduct the required development work in a professional manner, thus straddling the gap between research laboratory and clinic.

However, our endeavors to get research results out of the lab are not restricted solely to their translation into clinical applications. We are equally interested in the transfer of excellent ideas into products for commercial exploitation. Thus, science not

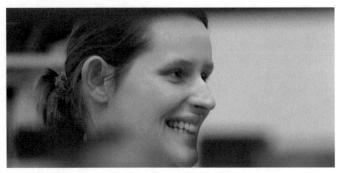

Marina Humburger, Division Molecular Biology of the Cell II

only fulfills its task of being a motor of economic development. By out-licensing our patents, we also try to make sure that promising approaches from research are turned into market ready products as swiftly as possible and, thus, become available for cancer patients all over the world. The article on page 160 describes the first hurdles that a potential compound from the German Cancer Research Center has to overcome on its way to the pharmacies.

Economic exploitation of results often requires close collaboration with industrial partners. Long-term partnerships are ideal to minimize friction in this cooperation between the two cultures of an industrial company and a research institute, for both sides need to

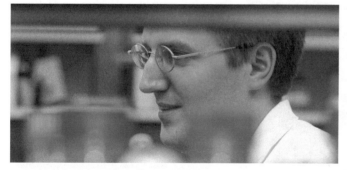

Sven Hoppe, Division Molecular Biology of the Cell II

learn about each other's needs and requirements. Thus, medical physicists of the German Cancer Research Center have been cooperating for many years with the company Siemens Medical Solutions in

the field of radiation therapy. The collaboration has already produced instrument prototypes and software for radiotherapy planning. The article on page 117 gives an account of this successful collaboration. By concluding a strategic alliance with Siemens in January 2006, we took our collaboration another step further: Both partners are combining their expertise in the field of radiological oncology in order to further develop integrated systems for imaging and radiation therapy. DKFZ scientists will have access to the latest instrument prototypes by Siemens including a 7-Tesla high-field magnetic resonance imaging system. In return, the German Cancer Research Center will provide its comprehensive scientific know-how to the industrial partner.

Despite all our efforts to translate our research into applications, we never lose sight of the fact that successful translation is always based on the results of excellent fundamental research.

Hence, the latter will continue to be a priority at the DKFZ. Numerous articles in this book give an impressive account of the excellent quality of research performed at the German Cancer Research Center.

Our Center is currently experiencing a time of change: Many scientific divisional heads are about to retire, including researchers who have helped to shape the face of the Center over many decades. In every change there is a chance: We have to continually re-adjust the scientific orientation of our Center. On the one hand, we have to invest in those areas where we already have a very good standing in the international scientific landscape in order to establish true "beacons" in these areas. Examples of such areas are apoptosis research and the development of radiotherapy methods, which are highlighted in the articles on pages 91 and 117. On the other hand, science continuously advances; new meth-

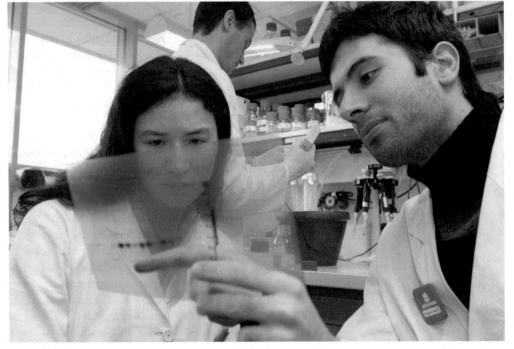

Andrea Perlewitz and Onur Cizmecioglu,
Research Group Mammalian Cell Cycle Control Mechanisms

Boveri Program as an instrument for supporting young scientists. In the meantime, more than a dozen independent young scientists' groups operate at our Center. It is our special concern to offer long-term professional prospects to excellent young working group leaders. Therefore, these positions are connected with a tenure track option following the American example, i.e., after positive evaluation of their work, the best junior researchers are given the opportunity to firmly establish a working group at the Center.

Support of young researchers at the DKFZ is not restricted to scientists who have completed their scientific training, it starts much earlier: The doctoral work is a crucial step in a young scientist's career, for this is often when the course is set for the rest of his or her professional life as a researcher. To help our roughly 350 doctoral students to complete their work within a reasonable time, with

ods and approaches lead to new questions, which enable us to reach new findings. Examples in the area of cancer research include epigenetics, systems biology, or the topic of cancer stem cells. To be able to respond with flexibility to such trends and to establish innovative research fields without delay at the DKFZ, we have attached great importance to young scientists' groups in recent years. For young scientists, the opportunity to establish their own independent working group early on is a crucial step in their career. A few years ago, the German Cancer Research Center took account of this by creating the Theodor

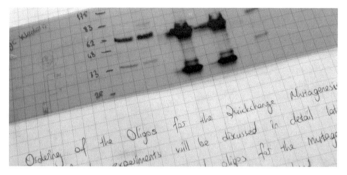

intensive supervision and extensive lecture courses, we have established a comprehensive training program. It was supplemented, in 2004, by the International PhD Program, which supports 36 excellent students from throughout the world each year. You will find more information about this program in the article on page 170.

In the long term, the innovative power of a society – and, of course, our survival as a research institute – depends on talented and committed young people taking up a career in science. To make sure that this source of young scientists does not dry up in the future, the German Cancer Research Center finances the Heidelberg Life Science Lab. This model program, which is conceivable only in a research environment such as Heidelberg, introduces school students from the 8th grade upwards to independent research projects which they can pursue at various institutes in Heidelberg. Read about the students' activities and projects on page 176.

We intend to take even more advantage in future of our excellent location in Heidelberg and the unique scientific environment it provides. A key objective of our collaborations with neighboring institutes such as the University Hospitals, the University, the Max Planck Institutes and the EMBL is to use synergy effects – both in terms of know-how transfer and optimized use of resources. Thus, we will continue to pursue our major goals in the years to come: to further expand our top international position in cancer research and to contribute results that help to diagnose cancer earlier, treat it successfully or prevent it, and to lessen human suffering.

Prof. Dr. Otmar D. Wiestler
Chairman of the Management
Board and Scientific Director of the
German Cancer Research Center

A Home for Research

It is impossible to overlook, and the noise broadcasts the news yet more forcefully: The Deutsches Krebsforschungszentrum (German Cancer Research Center, DKFZ) has turned into a huge building project. Our main building had come of age. Even though its external appearance may not have betrayed the fact, the state of the technical installations within left much to be desired: The multi-storied building was originally designed to accommodate a staff of 800, but of late there were at times as many as 1500 colleagues squashed into the main building and its extensions. The situation was no longer bearable for the staff, nor was it consistent with maintaining the quality of our

research. The technical infrastructure was worn out, the capacity of conduits was too low and no longer satisfied the high-tech demands of a modern laboratory operation. An insufficient heat shielding meant that in the summer months, especially in the south-facing laboratories, sensitive equipment frequently broke down due to overheating.

The extent of the renovation required had become so great that even complete demolition was considered. But this would have been a far more expensive solution, and furthermore, until such time as we could move into a new building, we could not have provided the neces-

sary alternative space for all members of staff. Thus it was decided to undertake a full-scale renovation whilst continuing to use the building. The work is not being carried out floor-by-floor but rather section-by-section from top to bottom, in each case over all eight floors, an approach that makes better technical and economic sense.

Once the project's funding was secured through our sponsors, the federal government and the State of Baden-Wuerttemberg, work began to plan the complex program of relocation, a logistic masterpiece of our Technical Services Division: Alternative premises were sought and found in Technol-

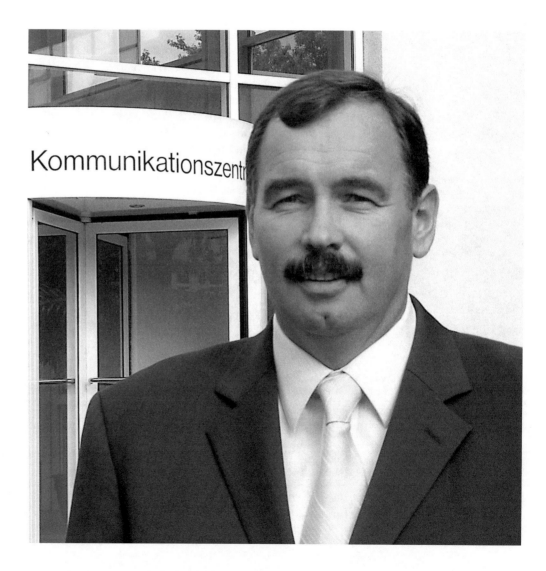

Dr. Josef Puchta, Administrative-
Commercial Director of the German
Cancer Research Center

ogy Park 4, where we were able to rent a space of about 5000 square meters. The preparation of a laboratory infrastructure in these alternative premises; the relocation of scientific divisions from the areas of the first section to undergo renovation; the successive relocation of further research groups into the newly renovated sections of the building, and the planning of the final allocation of premises once all the building work is finished – all these factors posed immense challenges for the organizers of this complex project.

The renovation is a burden to all the staff at the Center – whether through the hardship of having to move labs, or the noise and dust created by the building site in the next room or beneath one's window. There is hardly anyone who is not longing for the day – scheduled for the end of 2009 – when the work on the building will be completed.

In fact the renovation of our main building is only one of a number of building projects that are currently in progress. Soon we will begin the long overdue reconstruction and enlargement of our animal house. In the process of decoding the human genome, scientists discovered many genes whose role in the organism remained a mystery. To shed light on the function of these newly decrypted sections of genetic material, studies of genetically modified mice are indispensable. Hence our requirement for animal accommodation has increased significantly in recent

Cornelia Magin, Division Molecular Biology of the Cell II

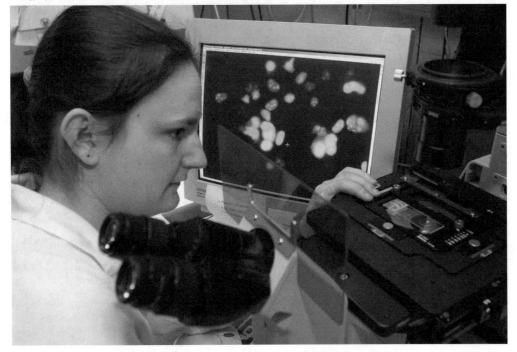

years. We will gain additional space by building three new stories onto our workshop block, so that when this is finished we can give up a few technically outdated laboratory containers used for animal housing. State of the art ventilation technology will make it possible to keep more mice per unit area in the new animal block and still ensure a germ-free environment, so that in future the risk of losing important breeding lines through virus infection will be minimized.

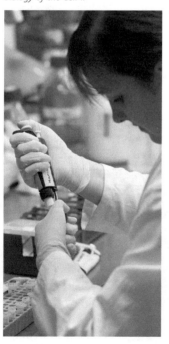

Marlene Roth, Division Molecular Biology of the Cell II

At the beginning of this year, the German Cancer Research Center was chosen in a competition of the Helmholtz Association to receive a new 7-Tesla high-field magnetic resonance imaging system. This is a piece of diagnostic equipment that promises to bring a whole new dimension to the temporal and spatial image resolution, right down to the level of individual molecules. With it, one should be able to determine the posi-

tion, extension, structure, blood supply, and metabolism of a tumor in far greater detail than has been possible up to now. However, the enormously high fields of the machine demand very substantial magnetic screening – for which more than 300 tons of steel are needed. Furthermore, the high-performance tomograph also requires a precise regulation of the air humidity and temperature. The only way to satisfy all these demands is to house the tomograph in its own specially constructed building. For this building, the university has generously provided us with a plot of land in our immediate neighborhood, which will facilitate the work of the radiologists.

Providing the scientists with an adequately equipped building is only one – albeit currently a very time-consuming one – of the tasks for which the administrative-commercial section of the DKFZ is responsible. The central mandate for the man-

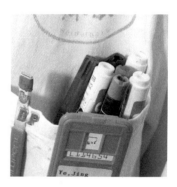

agement of a research institute is to acquire the necessary funding from public and private sources, to continuously improve the quality of the research facility, and to maintain and promote the creativity of the scientists by providing appropriate working conditions. Through the services provided in the sections Finance and Accounting, Personnel, Procurement, Administration of External Funding, and Technical Services we help the researchers to stay at the front in the international field of scientific competition. In turn, the high scientific reputation of the Center gives us an advantage in the competition to attract the best brains. Here too we have to judge ourselves and be judged according to international standards if we are to avoid losing our best scientists to institutes abroad.

In order to better judge our performance in this area, we decided to take a step which is routine in the research divisions of the Center, but which in the management field is still an exception: To undergo an evaluation by internationally renowned experts in the field of research management. The assessment board, comprising experts from economics and science, attested to the overall high quality of our work. The experts strengthened our resolve to increasingly orient ourselves towards the guidelines of the 'New Public Management': To move away from directive bureaucracy towards transparency, planned performance and targets, and attention to strategic aims. Overall, the evaluation made us aware of ways in which we can in future provide improved conditions for research and orient ourselves more efficiently towards the needs of our 'customers' – the scientists.

Management in science is not exclusively the domain of professional science managers. Successful young researchers in particular often find themselves, earlier than anticipated, in a situation in which they are expected to take on management duties: Responsibility

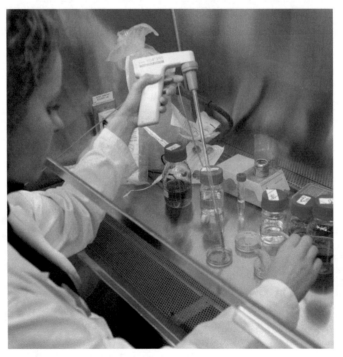

Cathleen Hanisch, Division Cell Biology

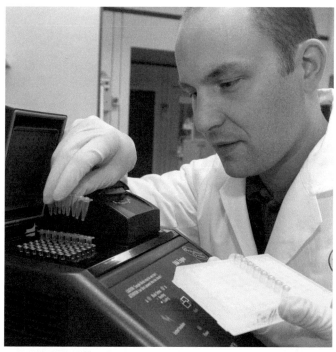

Daniel Habermehl,
Division Molecular Biology of the Cell I

for personnel, project management, coordination of international research projects – all these tasks arise at the latest when they begin to establish their own research group or division. In recent years, the research centers of the Helmholtz Association have been supporting the development of new junior research groups. At the German Cancer Research Center alone, more than a dozen new group leaders from the young generation have taken up positions since 2002. It is exactly these young colleagues who are often poorly prepared for their new management tasks. To improve this situation, the DKFZ has laid on more seminars and training courses. Furthermore, an Academy for Managers of the Helmholtz Association, the concept of which is currently being developed, is intended to teach the necessary soft skills and to provide the participants with the support of mentors who can give individual coaching. The training program will also be open to young managers from the infrastructure and administrative-commercial sections.

From the provision of technical facilities via improved communication structures to training in management skills – all these together yield the environment that we as management of a research center can create in order to promote the creativity and motivation of our scientists. Guidance by establishing an overall framework – this is the concept for keeping pace with the continual demand for change and adjustment that goes hand in hand with the enormous rate of progress in the life sciences. Only in this way can we contribute in the long term to maintaining the high scientific quality for which the German Cancer Research Center is known.

Dr. Josef Puchta
Administrative-Commercial
Director of the German Cancer
Research Center

The Research Programs

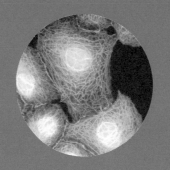

Research Program Cell Biology and Tumor Biology

Research is focused on cellular signaling pathways, which control almost all life processes: Growth and differentiation of the cell, embryo shape formation, or programmed cell death (apoptosis) are all regulated by cascades of biological signals. The signaling molecules can act on a cell from the outside, such as hormones, growth factors and inflammation mediators, or be produced by the cell itself. In response to the molecular message of these signaling cascades, genes in the nucleus of the recipient cell are eventually read or silenced. In this way, a cell initiates, for example, differentiation of a stem cell into a specialized tissue cell, starts an activation program or the release of hormones.

Researchers are investigating which defects in this cellular fine tuning can promote growth or cause resistance to death signals and, thus, lead to cancer. Genes controlling embryonic development also often play an important role in cancer development. Therefore, the

cellular signaling chains are also being investigated in embryos of model organisms such as Drosophila (fruit fly) and Xenopus (clawed frog).

Another research subject are the differences between normal and cancer cells in their architecture and equipment with transport molecules regulating the import and export of substances. A new research area deals with epigenetic changes of tumor cells that are potentially reversible and, thus, can be influenced using appropriate drugs.

Cancer cells are in a permanent exchange with their environment, especially with the connective-tissue stroma that surrounds and supports them. In recent years, it has become increasingly obvious that tumors cannot be regarded as isolated entities. Thus, under certain circumstances, tumor growth can be promoted by the stroma. A new approach in the development of cancer treatments is to interfere with these interactions.

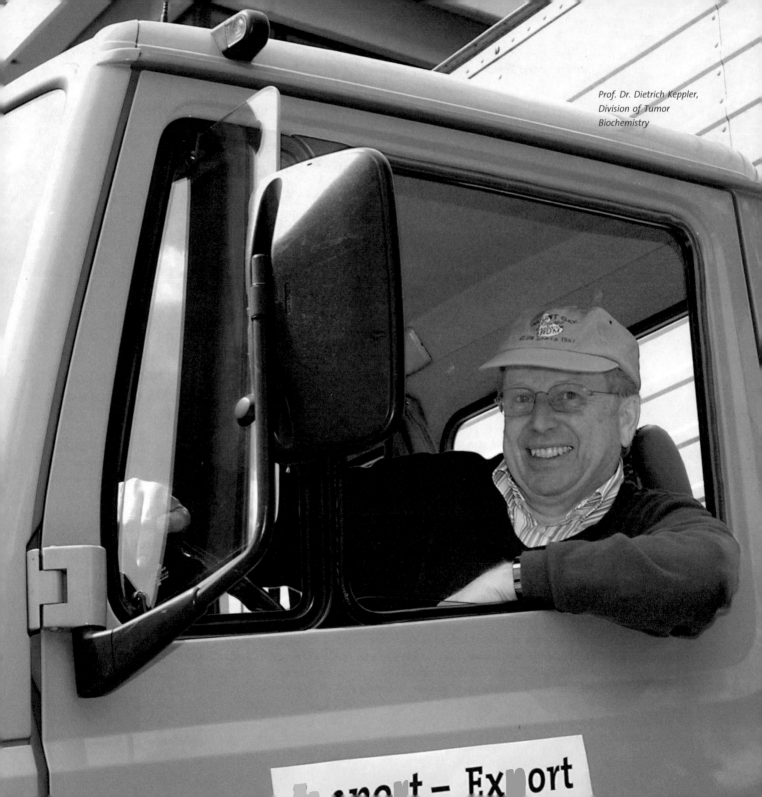

Prof. Dr. Dietrich Keppler,
Division of Tumor
Biochemistry

ort – Export

Import-Export across Cell Borders

Import proteins get substances into the cell; export pumps transport them back out. Hence the effectiveness of drugs also depends on a cell's equipment with these transport molecules

For much of his professional life, Dietrich Keppler has devoted himself to transportation. Up until recent years, he focused entirely on export; meanwhile he has started working in import, too. Professor Keppler's domain is not the shipping trade or the wholesale and export business. His shipments do not cross national borders, but the double lipid layer of biological cell membranes.

In 1973, biochemists obtained the first ever proof of a phenomenon that is today considered the most important mechanism in the development of resistances to cytostatic drugs used to treat cancer: Tumor cells increase the production of a membrane protein that acts like a pump. As soon as a cytotoxin arrives within a cell, it gets transported back out. Thus, the drug does not reach the required level and chemotherapy fails. The molecular pump, however, does not restrict its activity to the drug, but almost randomly transports other substances out of the cell. Meanwhile, a large variety of such multidrug resistance proteins are known, many of them are grouped under the term ABC transporters (see box on page 27).

Keppler, head of the Tumor Biochemistry Division, and his coworkers have invested more than a decade into studying these molecular transporters. They focused primarily on membrane pumps of the MRP family, today called ABCC proteins. Researchers of Keppler's division were able to elucidate the structure, localization, tasks, and substrate specificity of several members of the MRP family and to show their role in liver and renal cell cancers.

ABC transporters differ in their preferences for molecular cargo, although their specificities do overlap. In addition, not all transporters are present in all tissues. Keppler sees a chance here of making treatment decisions more specific in the future. His goal is to create a systematic catalogue of the transporter profiles of different tumors. "An unsuccessful chemotherapy is a double burden for patients: They have to endure severe side effects and they are losing valuable time. However, if we know the transporter equipment of the important tumors, we are able to avoid drugs that will in all probability provide no benefits for the patient."

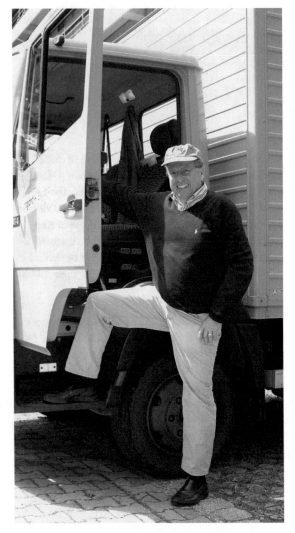

More Specific Chemotherapy to Treat Pancreatic Cancer

Keppler and his coworker, PD Dr. Jörg König, have started working on pancreatic cancer. The biochemists are collaborating in this project with physicians of the University Surgical Hospital Heidelberg. In Germany, tumors of the pancreas are the fourth most frequent cause of cancer death in women and the fifth most frequent cancer death in men. Sufferers usually survive only three to six months from the time of diagnosis. Pancreatic cancer is often not detected until it is too late for successful surgical removal and it is particularly resistant to chemotherapy.

The scientists found that several of the nine MRP transporters are not found in the pancreas at all, while others do not show any differences in expression between a healthy pancreas and a tumor. Production of MRP3 and MRP5, however, is increased up to ten times in carcinomas compared to a healthy pancreas – a strong indication that cytostatic drugs, which are among the substrates of these two pumps, are ineffective against the cancer. The researchers have devoted special attention to MRP3, whose level correlates with what is called tumor grading: The more typical characteristics of a pancreatic cell have been lost in a tumor cell – i.e., the more de-differentiated it is –, the more MRP it produces. The production increase is not a response to prior treatment with the substrates of this transporter, such as the cytostatic drug methotrexate. Instead, it is known that MPR3 plays a role in regeneration processes of the liver which involve de-differentialtion of hepatocytes. Apparently, MPR production is specifically boosted by the loss of differentiation.

In addition, the researchers recognized a relationship between MPR3 expression and disease progression: Patients whose MPR3 level in the tumor was below a certain threshold value had a significantly longer survival. Should this finding be confirmed, then MRP expression may be used in future by physicians as an indicator for individual prognosis and thus support the choice of appropriate treatment plans.

Import Proteins Provide Access to Cancer Cells

Some years ago, scientists still believed that cytostatic agents, most of which are fat-soluble, pass the cell membrane barrier simply by passive diffusion. Today, however, experts mostly agree that for the uptake of cytostatic drugs to be rapid enough, specific uptake transporters need to be involved. Thus, not only an excess of export pumps, but also a lack of specific uptake proteins can prevent that the required intracellular dose of cytotoxins is reached. In numerous tumors, researchers have discovered a group of import proteins called organic anion transporters (OATPs), which provide access to cells for a broad range of substances including various cytostatic drugs.

In the chemotherapy of brain tumors, cytotoxins have to overcome the blood-brain barrier before reaching

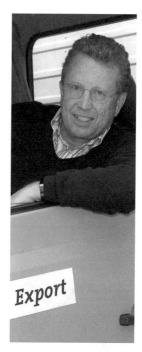

Dietrich Keppler investigates import and export of the cell

the tumor cell membrane. Gliomas, a common type of tumor, are particularly dreaded because of their strong chemoresistance. A detailed analysis of their membrane transporter equipment will help to find molecular loopholes through this double barrier. Jointly with doctors of the Neurosurgical University Hospital Heidelberg, Keppler and his coworker PD Dr. Anne Nies and Holger Bronger started a project to characterize the import/export profile of gliomas. The researchers used tissue samples from tumor surgery to determine the expression of six ABCC (the new term for MRP) transporters and six OATP transporters. Their investigation showed that ABCC4 and ABCC5 seem to be responsible for the export of a number of chemotherapy drugs in gliomas. It has been documented that ABCC4 mediates resistance to ganciclovir, methotrexate and topotecan.

The situation on the side of the import proteins, however, turned out to be more difficult. Thus, OATP1A2

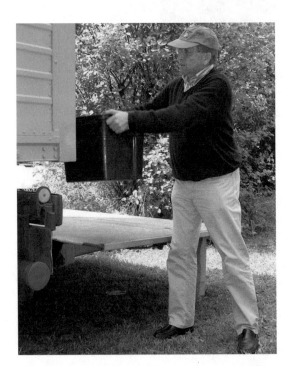

and OATP2B1 were found in the blood-brain barrier, but not in the membrane of the tumor cells. This explains the known failure of chemotherapy. The researchers do not yet exclude the possibility that import proteins of other families might help chemotherapy drugs access cancer cells. If not, then scientists see hardly any chance of success to cure gliomas using traditional chemotherapy.

Membrane Transport in the Culture Dish

Pharmacologists have begun to appreciate the significance of membrane transporters for the effectiveness of many drugs. Not only the chemotherapy of tumors depends on the import and export of substances; heart glycosides, inhibitors of cholesterol synthesis, or antiviral substances also need to reach certain effective levels. With a test to predict the "transportability" of new drugs, it would become possible to assess the chances of success of many substances already in an early stage of drug development.

Using his expertise in import/export matters, Keppler and colleagues were able to develop a test system that works with cells in a culture dish. The procedure, which has been designed also for semi-automated use, imitates a transport modality by which substances are moved through cellular layers: In many tissues of our body there are cavities and tubes sealing off an enclosed space from the "outside world". Examples include the intestinal lumen, the proximal kidney tu-

ATP Transporters

Following the discovery of the first molecular pump, mdr-1/P-glycoprotein, another group of membrane export proteins has been found since 1992: The MRP proteins (short for *multidrug resistance proteins*) mediate resistance to various structurally unrelated cytostatic drugs. Unlike mdr-1/P-glycoprotein, which transports fat-soluble substances out of the cell, the export mechanism of MRP proteins is based on a slightly more complicated mechanism, which was elucidated by Dietrich Keppler's coworkers in 1994: Lipophilic (water-insoluble) substances are first coupled in the cell to water-soluble, negatively charged molecules such as glutathione or glucuronic acid and then transported to the extracellular environment as conjugates.

Since all members of this transport protein family use the cellular power reserve, ATP, for their pumping activity and have structural characteristics in common, they are grouped under the term ABC transporters *ATP-binding cassette*). A total of 48 genes encoding for such molecular pumps have been identified in the human genome.

The physiological task of export pumps is to facilitate the release of endogenous substances and degradation products as well as exogenous toxic substances. Thus, in 1994, Keppler's division was able to show that MRP1 exports from mast cells, with high affinity, leukotriene C4, a key substance in the development of asthma and inflammatory reactions. ABC transporters are also responsible for the secretion of bilirubin and sexual hormone conjugates into the bile. Alongside their fatal role in the development of resistance of tumor cells, ABC transporters also serve cancer prevention. MRP2 discharges a number of food carcinogens into the intestinal lumen and also eliminates the fungal carcinogen aflatoxin B1 from hepatocytes. Thus, it is part of the body's own protection program against liver cell cancer.

bules, and the bile ducts. Cells that make up the border layers, or epithelia, have two sides with different functions. The apical (outward-facing) side is exposed to the "external environment" of the organ, i.e. the intestinal lumen or secretory tubules. The basolateral (inward-facing) side of the cell is in contact with the blood supply of the tissue. This type of cell architecture is called polar. The different functions of the apical and basolateral membranes are reflected in different protein make-ups. The passage of substances between polarized cells is prevented by special layers called tight junctions.

Substances to be transported outward from the bloodstream need to pass the polar epithelial cells. For this transcellular transport, the cells are equipped in the basolateral membrane with special uptake transporters such as those of the OATP family. By contrast, the apical membrane is equipped with export pumps, typically ABC transporters.

For his test system Keppler uses a cell line that is derived from dog kidneys and possesses only few transporter molecules of its own. These cells were additionally equipped with genes encoding for pairs of membrane transporters in humans: They were each supplied with one basolateral import protein and one apical export protein. Thus equipped, the cells are perfect models for molecular transport processes through a variety of human epithelia.

"A good example are statins", explains Dietrich Keppler. "They block cholesterol synthesis in liver cells. But to do so, they first have to get inside." Whether third-generation statins, which are currently being developed, succeed in doing so, is being investigated by many pharmaceutical companies using Keppler's double transfectant system. Keppler and his coworker Jörg König and Dr. Yunhai Cui recognized the application possibilities of the test in time and have obtained patent protection for the invention. Through license agreements, companies can use the DKFZ development for their research. There is hardly a leading pharmaceutical company today that does not use Keppler's system.

In the search for improved chemotherapies, researchers also expect much of the double transfectants: The discovery of the export pumps immediately raised hopes of "outsmarting" chemoresistance using inhibi-

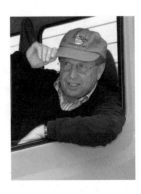

An expert in transport matters

tors of these molecules. The crux here is that the export inhibitors act only from inside – and rely on import transporters to do so. Many candidate inhibitors did not get past the testing stage; some acted so unspecifically that cell export came to a complete standstill. Many a substance has yet to be sent through the specially equipped canine kidney cells, before an enhanced substance will be found. There is no question that Keppler's test system will not run out of tasks in the near future.

Sibylle Kohlstädt

Literature

Bronger, H. et al.: Cancer Res. 65:1, 2005
König, J. et al.: Int. J. Cancer 115:359, 2005
Kopplow, K. et al.: Mol. Pharmacol. 68:1031, 2005

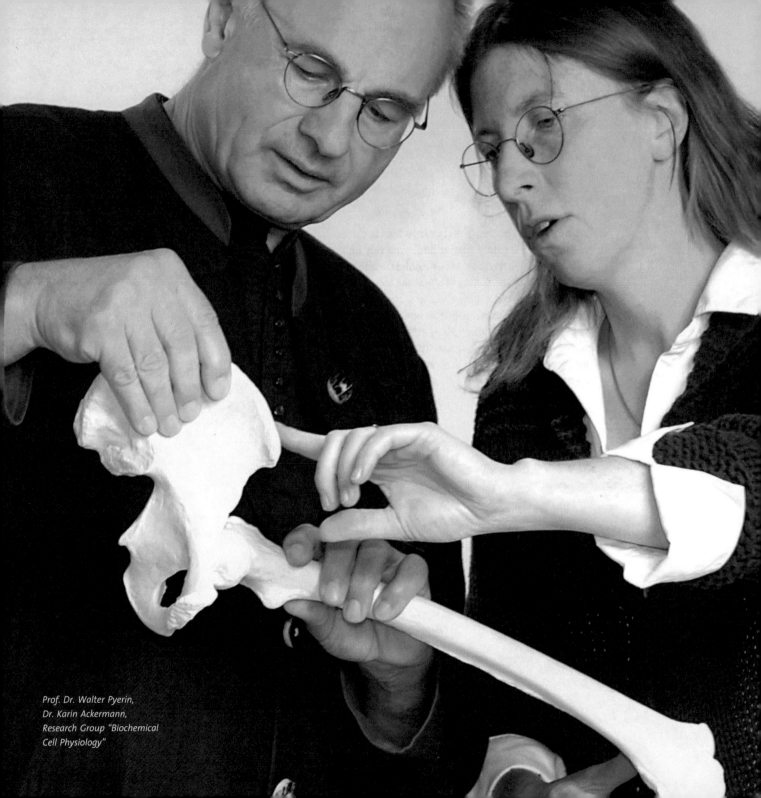

Prof. Dr. Walter Pyerin,
Dr. Karin Ackermann,
Research Group "Biochemical
Cell Physiology"

Camouflage Experts Beset Bone Cells

Migrated cancer cells make themselves invisible in the bone by adopting charac-teristics of their environment. A fatal co-existence where the bone helps meta-static tumor cells to settle down

Small hoverflies use this tactic, as do some butterfly species, snakes and fishes: They imitate the pattern and color of dangerous, poisenous or inedible species. Thus camouflaged, they are well protected against predators – a biological phenomenon called mimicry.

Cancer cells, too, are capable of adopting characteris-tics of other tissues. Disseminated cancer cells that co-lonize the bones as secondary tumors, or metastases, are particularly adept at camouflage: "They integrate themselves so well into the aggregate of bone cells that they are hardly distinguishable from these and they are also barely recognized by the immune sys-tem", explains Professor Walter Pyerin, head of the working group "Biochemical Cell Physiology", adding: "This is why we speak of osteomimicry."

Bone metastases are a major problem in prostate and breast cancers, but also in tumors of the lung and other organs. They frequently form at an early stage of the cancer – sometimes even before the primary tu-mor has been detected. Once the disseminated cells have colonized the bone tissue, they disrupt its deli-cate balance. After all, our skeleton is not made of stiff, liveless material. Instead, it is constantly being restructured as a result of the interplay of various types of bone cells – bone-forming osteoblasts and bone-resorbing osteoclasts (see box on page 34). Well-camouflaged disseminated cancer cells that invade bone disturb the continuous process of bone forma-tion and resorption. The result is disproportionate bone loss or gain – technically called local osteolytic or osteoblastic bone lesions – and severe, almost un-bearable pain.

Large-Scale Search in the Bone

"We have made it our goal to find out the mecha-nisms invading cancer cells use to make themselves invisible in the bone", says Pyerin's coworker, biologist Dr. Karin Ackermann, describing her project. Using this knowledge, the researchers hope to identify potential targets for treating the painful metastatic tumors.

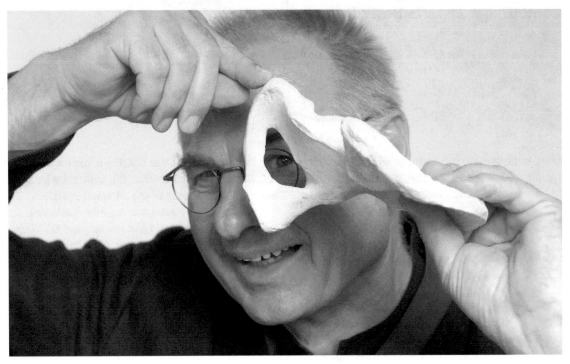

Pyerin and Ackermann have found first important evidence of how and why osteomimicry works using gene expression analyses. To this end, they applied microarray technology (also called DNA chip technology), a method that enables researchers to gain insight into gene activity on a large scale. Using small glass or nylon slides, it is possible to study several thousand genes in a single run. Expression chips are loaded with single-stranded DNA fragments called probes which serve to detect messenger RNA (mRNA) in sample material. Determining the type and number of mRNA molecules in a tissue provides information about which genes are active and their level of activity in a tissue. Conspicuous findings are subsequently verified at the protein level.

To investigate whether expression patterns of migrated cancer cells change in their new environment, the Heidelberg scientists copied the situation in the lab. They cultivated prostate cancer cells and bone

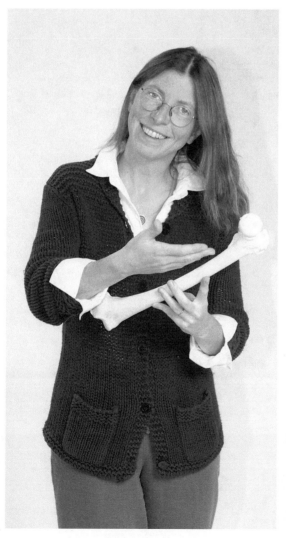

cells (bone-forming osteoblasts, to be precise) in the same culture dish. Separated by a fine screen, the different cell types had no direct contact with each other, but they were able to exchange their messenger substances via the culture medium.

A Fatal Dialogue

And really, after just one day the investigators noticed first peculiarities in the expression patterns of the cancer cells. Suddenly, genes became active that did not match the tissue type of origin – in this case the prostate –, but were typical of bones instead. Before long, it became clear that the osteoblasts in the culture dish send out signal molecules that eventually lead to alterations in the cancer cells. These partially adopt bone cell character. A fatal collaboration indeed, in which the bone first helps metastases to settle down, just to get destroyed by these. Thus, the invading transformed cells manage to attach themselves to their new environment, develop a striking resemblance to their new "neighbors" and become less noticeable for the immune system. "To date, we have identified several signal molecules that play a key role in this dialog between the two cell types", says Pyerin.

Thus, as a result of contact with the osteoblasts, a developmental control gene called sonic hedgehog becomes active in tumor cells. Normally, this gene is hardly ever read in adult tissue. The product of sonic

Anything But Stiff and Lifeless

At first sight, bone seems to be a lifeless, stiff scaffold. After all, it is not elastic, but breaks when we fall awkwardly. But the fact that such a broken bone grows back together shows: This is active body tissue. Due to a continuous process of bone formation and resorption, ten years from now none of our bones will be made up of the same substance as today.

Three cell types were identified as helpers in this process: Osteoblasts act relatively close to the surface. They permanently build bone by secreting components of the bone matrix, a layer that connects the different bone cells. This bonding material is elastic at first, but is soon turned into hard bone matrix due to calcium phosphate deposition. During this process, the osteoblasts get embedded and turn into star-shaped osteocytes connected among each other via long extensions. This type of cell produces only little material itself, but is still involved, through secretion of various signal molecules, in regulating bone formation and resorption. Finally, there are the osteoclasts which, as counterparts of the osteoblasts, resolve bone matrix – a process that is necessary to facilitate, for example, growth of blood vessels in growing bones. Migrating cancer cells colonizing this environment fatally disrupt this delicate balance. Crosstalk, i.e., signal exchange between bone cells and metastatic tumor cells, leads to a number of changes in gene expression on both sides. Among others, a gene is activated that encodes the information for a molecule named RANKL (receptor activator of NFκB-ligand) – a key player in the development of osteoporosis. This molecule attaches itself to a receptor (RANK) on the surface of osteoclasts, which are thus activated and start resolving bone substance. Simultaneously, the counteracting protein osteoprotegerin, which blocks RANKL in healthy bone, is downregulated so that this protection mechanism fails.

hedgehog triggers a signaling cascade in tumor cells and possibly in osteoblasts, too. This reaction chain leads to the production of bone morphogenic protein 2 (BMP2), which plays a key role in bone formation. In tumor cells, but additionally also in osteoblasts, BMP2 activates transcription factors that initiate the production of bone-forming proteins.

Individual steps of such activation chains may be suitable targets for therapy development. If these chains can be interrupted, it might be possible to prevent the nidation of secondary tumors. The team of the working group "Biochemical Cell Physiology" is currently conducting experiments with several substances designed to inhibit the effect of sonic hedgehog directly at the site of metastasis.

But the investigators observed even more changes in the cells in the culture dish. It became apparent that, reversely, cancer cells have a strong influence on gene expression of osteoblasts. Thus, in the bone cells there was an increased activity of a number of genes that play a role in the development of pain. These include, for example, genes that are responsible for the synthesis of mediator molecules such as prostaglandins.

Taking a Look into the Bone

So much for the culture dish. But do these observations correlate with actual processes in the body? To find out, Pyerin and Ackermann, jointly with their co-workers, have designed a method for investigating bone cells without disrupting the biochemical situation of a living organ. Using this method, the scientists have started to take a close look at tissue samples obtained from patients of Heidelberg and Mannheim University Hospitals. Once more they applied chip technology to compare gene expression of healthy bone fragments colonized by metastases.

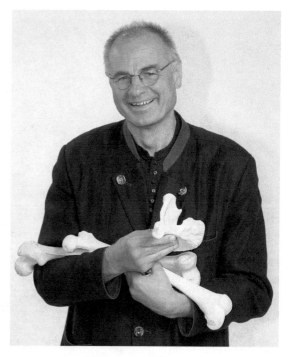

Once more, it turned out that the migrated cancer cells have an influence on which genetic information is read and transcribed into proteins. Gene expression in the osteocytes was found to be noticeably changed. In this most common cell type of the bone, the dialog with the metastases leads to the activation of a number of genes whose products are involved in processes such as building and maintaining cell structure or play a role in cell metabolism. In addition, like in the culture dish, genes became active whose products are associated with pain development. The candidate genes are currently being studied in further experiments. However, it is already becoming apparent that the bone cells themselves, due to their new "residents", undergo changes that might cause them to send out pain signals. This would mean that osteocytes, too, are involved in pain development; so far, researchers had assumed that only the colonizing metastases are responsible for this. This could provide explanations for previously uninterpretable pain patterns.

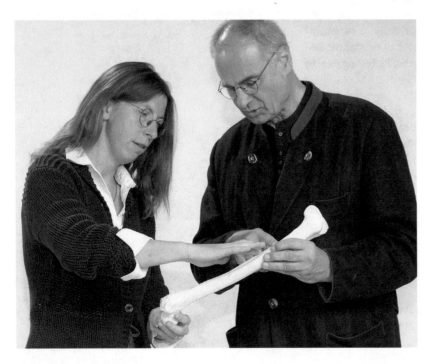

Cancer cells change gene expression in bone tissue

A Step Towards Diagnostics

But this is not all: Analysis of bone samples from patients with different cancers revealed that it is always the same genes – about one hundred altogether – whose activity is strikingly altered. These genes can be related to quite a variety of different cellular processes. Very surprisingly for the researchers, this does not always happen according to the same pattern, but there appear to be typical expression signatures. Thus, the activity of a particular gene can be reduced in metastases of breast cancer, while it is significantly increased in multiple myeloma – or vice versa. This shows that the tumor cells seem to leave a very specific molecular fingerprint in the osteocytes.

"We are observing these differences with such a constancy that we are convinced that one day we will be able to use this knowledge in cancer diagnostics", Ackermann says, assessing the relevance of this observation with a view to the future. For it isn't rare that elderly people are treated unsuccessfully for primary osteoporosis. The reason is that they really suffer from osteopathy caused by hardly detectable bone metastases. In such cases, analysis of selected marker genes whose activity is typically changed in bone metastases might lead to improved diagnosis and, thus, more successful treatment.

Stefanie Reinberger

Literature

Knerr, K. et al.: Int. J. Cancer 111:152, 2004
Eisenberger, S. et al.: Analyt. Biochem. 335:260, 2004
Neidhart, T. et al.: submitted

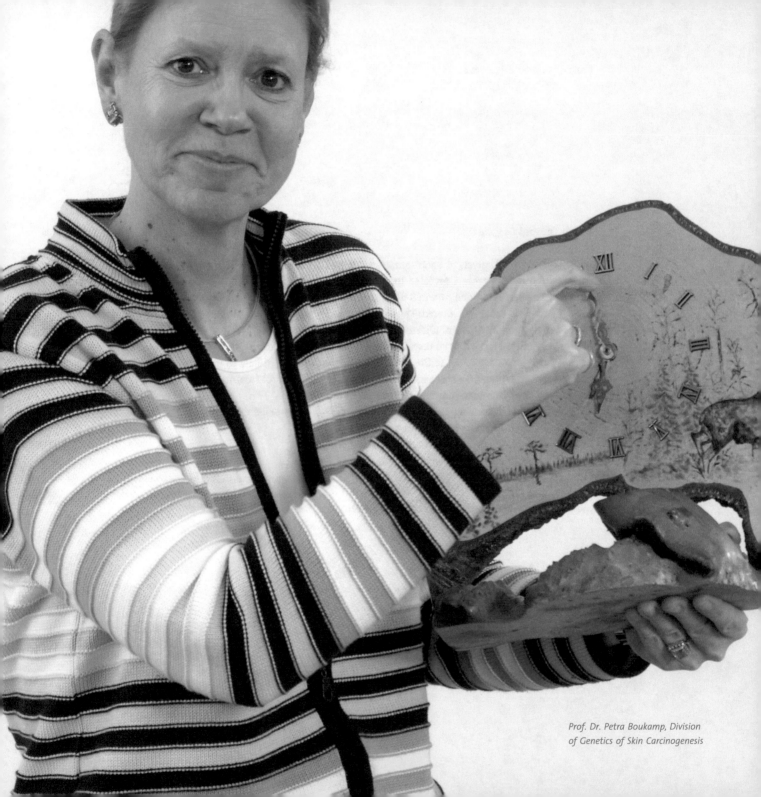

Prof. Dr. Petra Boukamp, Division
of Genetics of Skin Carcinogenesis

The Dance of the Telomeres

Protective caps at the chromosome tips: The function of telomeres goes far beyond that of a biological clock

"The cell's inner clock" or "immortality enzyme" – telomeres and telomerase have been dubbed with a variety of such names in the press. The true story of these chromosome end structures and the enzyme that keeps them intact is being investigated by Professor Petra Boukamp and her division. The primary aim of her research is to understand the role played by these components of the cell in the occurrence of cancer.

Regarded in molecular biological terms, the telomere amounts to a thousand-fold repetition of a particular DNA sequence, consisting of only six building blocks. These chromosome ends, however, do not exist simply as a linear succession of bases, they form a loop. This ensures that telomere ends cannot join onto one another, as would happen with certainty were it not for this protective structure. The telomeres function as a kind of protective cap, which prevents the genetic material from being damaged by the degrading enzymes known as exonucleases.

The Cell's Hourglass

An important function that is attributed to the telomere is that of a biological clock. Each time a cell divides the chromosome ends become somewhat shorter, and the protective cap thereby ever thinner. This continues until the cap reaches a critical lower limit. Then the cell receives the signal to stop dividing, whereupon it eventually dies. One speaks of cell aging. For the germline or for tissue that is continually renewing itself such as the blood-forming system, the skin, or the lining of the gut, nature has come up with a special solution: The enzyme telomerase works to prevent the degradation of the chromosome caps and allows the life-clock of the cells to keep ticking.

'Immortality enzyme' was what an American researcher called telomerase, because of its ability to keep cells alive indefinitely – at least in a culture dish. However, the Heidelberg scientist Boukamp is far from agreeing with this description. For this name is virtually a promise of eternal youth, whereas the overzealous telomerases are not something to play

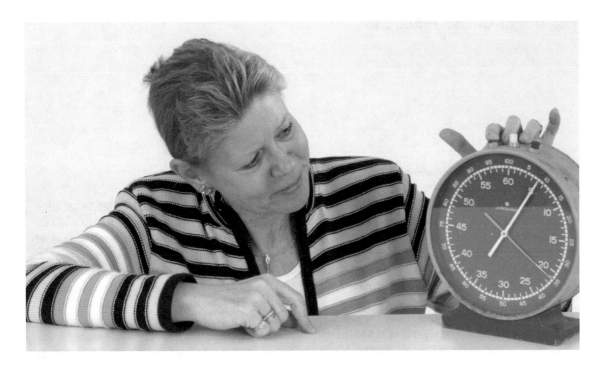

games with. Normally they should only be active in cells with a high frequency of division. In fully differentiated tissue, on the other hand, the enzyme is generally inactive. However, if in such cells it is switched on or up-regulated due to faulty control, the situation rapidly gets out of hand. The result can be a multiplication of cells and the development of tumors.

In fact we know that telomerase is active in about 90 per cent of all tumors. For this reason cancer researchers now believe that the enzyme is an important prerequisite for the uncontrolled multiplication of transformed cells. Substances that inhibit the activity of the telomerase and thus lead to a cessation of growth therefore offer a novel approach to cancer therapy. Clinical studies with such substances are already underway in the USA.

Short Ends Arouse Suspicion

Boukamp's view, however, is that such attempts are premature. "We know far too little about the way in which telomeres and telomerase work to intervene at such a profound level in the cellular processes", she says assertively and continues: "The possible consequences of such a therapy are currently completely unforeseeable." Her own investigations make clear that the enzyme is obviously needed in normal skin. This can be deduced from, among other things, skin samples from young test persons, about 30 years of age, which already display very short telomeres. The epidermis of the skin renews itself every four weeks. This means that skin cells must divide very frequently for a whole lifetime, their telomeres becoming shorter each time. Without telomerase, this continual cell division would have devastating consequences: Growth would stop prematurely, and the skin would very soon no longer be able to fulfill its function as an external shield. This shows clearly that for patients in a certain risk group – namely, those who already have short telomeres – medication to inhibit telomerase would be associated with the danger of damaging healthy tissue.

For the scientists in the Division "Genetics of Skin Carcinogenesis" one thing is for sure: Before risking trials of such therapies, there is still a huge amount to be learned about the chromosome caps and how they function. As a step in this direction, the team of re-

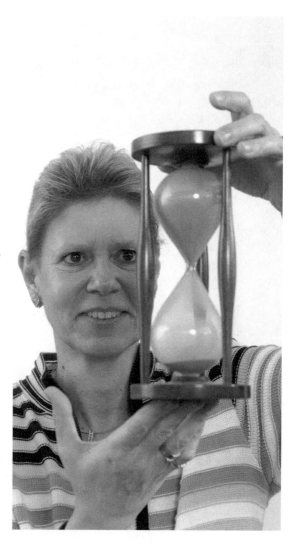

Hazardous Sunlight

Sunlight not only has a positive effect on the mood, it is of vital importance in enabling our bodies to produce the essential vitamin D. Nonetheless, it should be treated with the greatest respect, because UV light, to which we expose ourselves every time we bask in the sun or go to the solarium, is one of the leading environmental carcinogens. It is the cause of 90 percent of all cases of skin cancer.

Too much sun quickly makes itself felt – often in a painful way. If a certain maximum amount, which varies from one individual to another, is exceeded, the result is sunburn. For this the main culprit is UV-B.

But UV radiation also leaves traces in the genetic material. A typical example of damage are the so-called thymidine dimers: Two thymidine building blocks that neighbor one another on a DNA strand can, under the influence of UV-B irradiation, become firmly paired with one another. Provided the damage is not too extreme, the cell is able to defend itself. Special repair enzymes recognize the dimers and cut them out. The gaps that are left are filled up and the damage is removed. But beware – if the damage is extensive enough the repair troops cannot work fast enough and some of the dimers are overlooked. The remaining paired thymidines are no longer recognized as the original thymidine elements. Next time the DNA replicates prior to a cell division this produces reading errors, or mutations, which in turn can be at the root of a cancer.

Unlike the UV-B light, the UV-A component of the sunlight produces no damage at the level of the individual genetic building blocks. Rather – as can be deduced from the latest results of the Genetics of Skin Carcinogenesis Division at the German Cancer Research Center – UV-A contributes to the occurrence of tumors through its effects on chromosome stability.

How then should one exploit the positive effects of sunlight without risking massive damage and even skin cancer? The clear answer is: Protection against UV radiation with clothes or sun creams with a high protection factor (at least 15), in particular for children. Furthermore, it is advisable to avoid the sun during the midday period from 11 am to 3 pm, when the radiation is at its strongest. As an additional measure, clothes with special UV protection are sensible in some circumstances. Some modern sun creams, available in pharmacies, contain not only UV filters but also the enzyme photolyase, found in algae. It is supposed to help in repairing first DNA damage in the skin. The photolyase recognizes the thymidine dimers typical for UV damage and sticks to them; in doing so it breaks the bonds holding the two bases together.

searchers has developed a method for examining the effect of UV light on the length and distribution of telomeres in small skin samples.

Choreography of the Chromosome Ends

Petra Boukamp's team, working in close cooperation with colleagues in Canada, has succeeded for the first time in recording the spatial distribution of telomeres over the course of the reproduction cycle of a cell. Depending on the phase of the cell cycle, the DNA in the cell nucleus exists in different forms. In the resting and growth phases G_0 and G_1, for example, the chromosomes are relatively loosely distributed. In contrast, in the G_2 phase, shortly before the cell divides, and also during the division itself, they are highly organized and always follow the same paths through the nucleus. Only in this way can it be ensured that in the end both daughter cells possess the complete hereditary information.

But how do the telomeres behave during the various phases of the cell cycle? To get to the bottom of this question, Boukamp and her colleagues marked the chromosome ends with a fluorescent dye and followed the movements of the optical signals with the help of high-resolution microscopy and reconstruction of the telomeres in three dimensional space. It emerged that during the life cycle of the cells studied, the telomeres too follow a predetermined choreography. In the G_2 phase, for example, shortly before divi-

sion, they gather together in a characteristic disc-shaped formation, known in specialist jargon as the 'telomeric disc'.

A comparison of healthy with transformed cells revealed an amazing fact: In a few cancer cells the arrangement of the telomeres was severely disrupted. Instead of the well sorted distribution, here the scientists found downright clumps of telomeres, known as telomere aggregates. In the cancer cells some of the

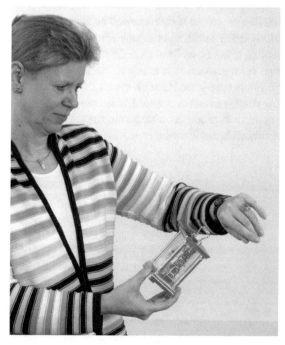

chromosome ends had obviously stuck together – exactly the state of affairs that the telomeres are intended to prevent.

Oncogene Promotes Telomere Aggregation

What then is the significance of these peculiar clumps? Do cancer promoting mechanisms influence the dance of the telomeres, or perhaps even destroy it? To answer this question, the Heidelberg team of researchers chose a cell line for closer examination. The cell line concerned is characterized by having too much active c-myc, an oncogene whose cancer promoting effect arises from its ability to stimulate massive cell reproduction. It is indeed the active c-myc which, in a very specific way, causes the formation of the strange telomere clumps noticed previously by the scientists in cancer cells. Moreover, the aggregates evidently alter the structure of some chromosomes. With-

in the clumps the chromosomes come into such close proximity that they can exchange individual sections with one another. This phenomenon is known as chromosome translocation.

This clearly demonstrates that cancer-causing mechanisms such as active c-myc have a decisive influence on the stability of chromosomes, and hence on that of the entire genome. The translocations change the arrangement of the hereditary material, which can lead to the activation of genes that give the cells a growth advantage. This, in consequence, facilitates a further transformation of the cells. Through their investigations, Boukamp and her cooperation partners have identified a completely new mechanism that can contribute to the development of cancer.

In their most recent experiments the researcher and her team found that too much UV radiation has a similar effect on the arrangement of the telomeres as the oncogene c-myc. In irradiated cells, too, the protective caps regularly stick together and arrange themselves into clumps. "In the meantime we know that the altered chromosomes and the associated causation of tumors are a consequence of these telomere aggregates", says Boukamp, summarizing the significance of her discovery. She continues: "And so our next aim will be a detailed study of the role of UV radiation in the formation of the clumps." Thereby she is referring in particular to the light produced by sun beds, the UV-A radiation.

In addition, the scientists want to investigate in detail whether the formation of aggregates produces further damage to the heredity material, over and above that due to chromosome translocation. One could imagine, for example, that after a cell division there might be an unequal distribution of the genetic material. "This sticking together might mean that, during mitosis, in which normally a full set of chromosomes finds its way into each daughter cell, some chromosomes end up on the wrong side", explains Boukamp. The consequence would be some cells in which chromosomes are duplicated, and others where they are missing – a state that is often observed in tumors. Thanks to this new knowledge gained by the Division of Genetics of Skin Carcinogenesis, it is becoming ever clearer that

the UV-A light can unleash devastating disorder in our cells, a state of chaos that can eventually lead to cancer. Petra Boukamp shakes her head as she concludes her explanation: "Knowing what we now know, it is hard to stand by and watch so many people frying themselves for hours in the sun or the solarium, or even allowing their children to play outside with no protection from the sun."

Stefanie Reinberger

Literature

Chang, T.C.Y. et al.: BMC Biology 2:12, 2004
Ermler, S. et al.: Europ. J. Cell Biol. 83:681, 2004
Louis, S.F. et al.: PNAS 102:9613, 2005

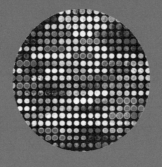

Research Program Structural and Functional Genomics

Cancer arises when the genetic material is changed in such a way that it causes the cell to divide in an uncontrolled manner. For this to happen, a multitude of specific changes have to coincide. It is the task of this Research Program to analyze the genome, i.e., the complete set of genes, in order to lay the foundation for developing new diagnostic and treatment methods. This involves mapping the genome, localizing genes within the genetic material, and analyzing the number and structure of chromosomes both in healthy and transformed cells.

Comparing the activity of individual genes and whole genomes of healthy cells and of tumor cells, researchers have also found significant differences that can be summarized into specific activity patterns. Scientists are searching for patterns which allow predictions about the prognosis or treatment response of tumors.

Another task of the Research Program is to develop high-throughput technologies that facilitate such studies of genes and gene activities on a large scale. The aim is to speed up the process of identifying and evaluating potential new target structures for cancer diagnosis and treatment. To handle the vast amounts of data accumulated in the process, the bioinformatics-oriented divisions of the Research Program are developing special biomathematical methods and models.

The second area of the Research Program consists of divisions that use approaches from mathematics, statistics, physics, computer sciences, and systems biology to develop computer-assisted simulation and modeling methods which make it possible to analyze the three-dimensional structure of the genome and biological macromolecules and to visualize metabolic processes in living cells.

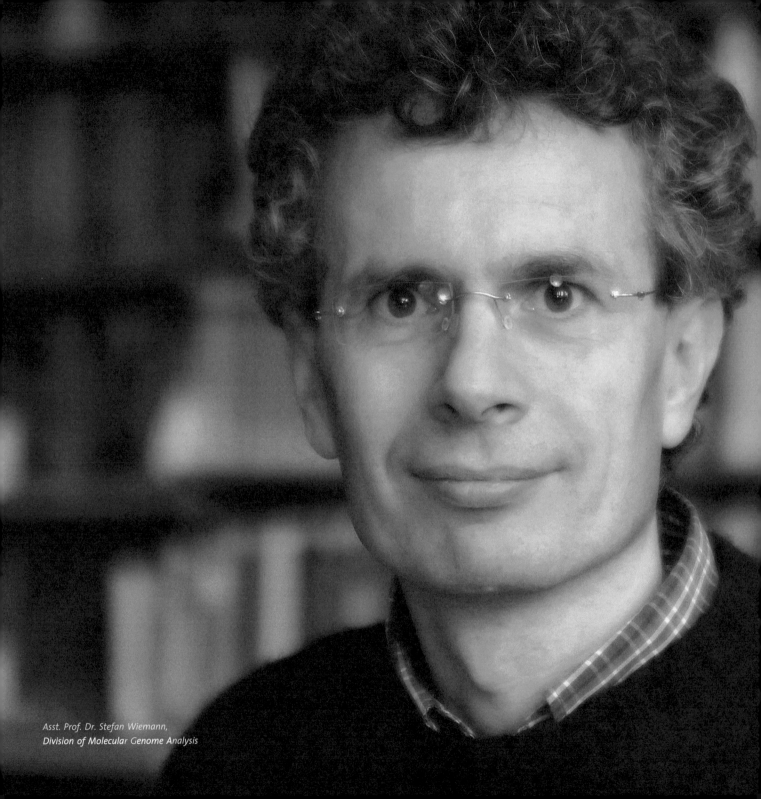

Asst. Prof. Dr. Stefan Wiemann,
Division of Molecular Genome Analysis

Assembly-Line Testing of Protein Functions

The German cDNA Consortium systematically investigates the functions and cellular localizations of all human proteins

It was one of the great media events of 2001: In a dramatic race, Craig Venter's company, Celera Genomics, competed with the public funded international Human Genome Project to publish the first ever "draft" version of the human genome sequence. Eventually, both versions were published at the same time. Only recently, in Spring 2005, the Human Genome Project published a completed and revised version of the sequence comprising roughly three billion base pairs.

Does that mean that man has uncovered every secret of the human genetic material? What does the genome tell us about genes, i.e., those one to two percent of DNA that are building instructions for proteins? No life without proteins: As enzymes they do all the metabolic work; as membrane receptors they regulate the complex processes of intercellular and intracellular communication; as components of the cytoskeleton they provide shape and support to the cell; as antibodies they protect the organism from pathogens. A defect in the base sequence of a gene leads to a defect in the protein. And almost always it is defects in protein functioning that cause human diseases.

Today, there are computer algorithms to find the protein encoding parts of the genome rather reliably. But the bare sequence of bases of genomic DNA does not always help to answer questions about the functions of individual proteins. Not even known yet is the exact number of protein encoding genes in the human genome. Although researchers all over the globe have been busy studying thousands of individual proteins, what was missing was a systematic search for yet unidentified proteins at the technical scale of the Human Genome Project.

"When we started the project, our aim was to capture the genetic information about protein structures in libraries. Only instead of books, these libraries contain cDNA clones", PD Dr. Stefan Wiemann explains. Wiemann is a molecular biologist who has been working at the Division of Molecular Genome Analysis headed by Professor Annemarie Poustka since 1995. cDNA is an artificial product that serves as an information carrier for molecular biologists studying proteins (see box on page 51). "We are not talking here about analyzing 20 or 30 cDNAs", says Wiemann looking back at the situation at the time. "We were thinking of orders of several hundred thousands!" There was no way for him and his then team of five to do this alone. In order to distribute the monstrous project onto several shoulders, the scientists initiated the formation of the German cDNA Consortium back in 1997. Alongside DKFZ , there are two other Helmholtz Centers in the consortium: the Munich-based National Research Center for Environment and Health (GSF) and the Gesellschaft für Biotechnologische Forschung (GBF) in Braunschweig. Another member based in Heidelberg is the European Molecular Biology Laboratory (EMBL).

Scientists of the consortium have produced about 560,000 cDNA clones to date. The next step was one of laborious work. The cDNAs had to be deciphered letter by letter. But why determine the sequence

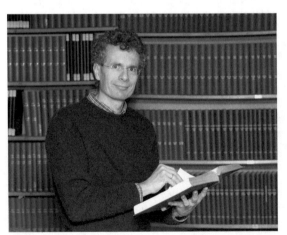

again, when it is already available in the data of the Human Genome Project? Because often, the protein encoding sequence has only little in common with the DNA sequence from the nucleus. Many processing steps within the cell trim the protein information; sometimes totally different proteins are read from one and the same DNA segment by different processing.

About 230,000 clones have been partially sequenced; several thousand of these contain the protein information in full length. In total, the cDNA Consortium has labored through 50 million base pairs. The sequence information is made universally accessible through EMBL's database. In addition, the Resource Center for Genome Research makes cDNA clones available to scientists and companies to conduct their own research.

Identifying Localizations

A first clue about a protein's possible task is its localization within the cell. A protein that is anchored exclusively in the cell membrane is not able to do any work in the nucleus. However, a protein that dwells in the mitochondria, may well be involved in the cellular power supply.

Jointly with researchers at EMBL, Wiemann's team started an ambitious project: the systematic identification of the localizations of as yet undescribed proteins. To this end, cDNAs are introduced in cells in the cul-

The Magic Word is cDNA

All protein encoding genes in a cell are first copied, i.e. an RNA transcript is generated. During this process, portions of a gene with no protein information, called introns, are removed. In addition, a specific recognition label called poly-A tail is added to the end of each transcript. The poly-A tail is a long, monotonous stretch of adenosine bases. For molecular biologists, it is gift of nature because it provides them with an ideal tool for isolating the messenger RNA molecules from the cell lysate. Using an enzyme known as reverse transcriptase, these are then transcribed back into DNA. DNA molecules thus generated are called cDNA (c for copy), because they are an exact copy of the messenger RNA. Introduced into cells or bacteria, the cDNA serves as a template used by the organism's protein synthesis apparatus to produce the respective protein. A bacterial colony in a Petri dish which multiplies a specific cDNA molecule is technically called a clone.

ture dish. Before doing so, they are labeled with the jellyfish's GFP protein, which fluoresces green under the microscope. Thus, it is possible to see at a glance in which area of the cell proteins settle down after being synthesized.

About one thousand cDNAs have been categorized in this way on the basis of their cellular localization. Systematic use of life cell imaging, a type of video image that captures even intracellular dynamics, promises to yield even more detailed information.

To provide access to this information for the international scientific community, the Heidelberg scientists created an Internet database. At www.dkfz.de/LIFEdb, researchers from all over the world can obtain pictures of protein localizations – combined with all other data on a particular cDNA that have been gathered so far.

Alongside the German cDNA Consortium, two other large-scale cDNA projects have been started in the world: the U.S. Mammalian Gene Collection and an association of Japanese researchers. Their common goal is to identify all human genes and make these available in the form of cDNA clones. Since 2002, researchers from these three projects have held regular big workshops where the international cDNA community comes together to relate all information gathered so far to the respective cDNAs: sequence data, alternative splicing isoforms, functional domains, polymorphisms, gene expression profiles, subcellular localizations,

matches with mouse gene sequences. More than
41,000 cDNAs have already been fed into the jointly
operated H-Invitational Database, which can be ac-
cessed on the Internet at http://www.h-invitatio-
nal.jp/.

Functional Testing in the Thousands

The whereabouts of a protein molecule is only a first
hint about its possible function or disease relevance.
Further tests are required to answer these questions.
However, as in the localization tests before, scientists
are encountering a problem here: By introducing
cDNA into cells, these are forced, so to speak, to produce the respective protein – often at levels that have
nothing in common with the natural situation. At-
taching the fluorescent jellyfish protein might also influence their behavior. Stefan Wiemann explains: "We

These are books.
But Stefan Wiemann's libraries contain cDNA clones

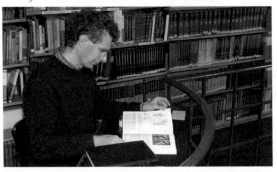

have to take special care here: We chiefly observe
those cells that express small amounts of the proteins
and we also perform cross-checks: Using RNAi technology, a way of blocking protein expression, we study
what happens if we selectively reduce production of
the protein of interest. Moreover, we attach the GFP
marker to both ends of the protein and check whether
this leads to different localizations or effects."

Now scientists are spoilt for choice: Which of the
many thousand cDNAs to select for functional tests?
Selection is necessary because they are interested first
and foremost in proteins that are linked to diseases.
At the German Cancer Research Center this would be
primarily cancer. In this respect, Wiemann gets support from his colleague, PD Dr. Holger Sültmann, who
leads the working group "Gene Expression in Tumors"
in Poustka's division. Sültmann has been studying the
genetic material of various healthy and malignant
cells on DNA microarrays. In the process, he identifies
all those genes that are read more or less in transformed cells compared to normal ones and, thus, seem
to be linked to cancer in some way or other. This information helps Wiemann to concentrate his functional tests on promising candidates.

The functional protein analysis research performed by
the Heidelberg researchers is embedded in a network
of research projects that jointly form the "Systematic
Methodological Platform (SMP) Cell", a module of the
National Genome Research Network. The SMP Cell has
committed itself to the systematic investigation of the

cDNA resources generated by the Consortium to search for links to important diseases (see box on page 54). The work is distributed according to the specialist expertise of the participating institutes; Stefan Wiemann is the coordinator.

Functional analysis at the DKFZ is focused on tests which give information about a protein's involvement in cellular processes that typically get out of control

in cancer. For example, scientists are studying caspase 3 activation to find out whether this candidate induces apoptosis, i.e. programmed cell death, in cells. Incorporation of BrdU, a substance that is an analog of DNA building blocks, into cellular DNA is a signal of DNA synthesis, i.e., the cell starts dividing. Activation of MAP kinases by an unknown protein under investigation also indicates a role in cell proliferation and differentiation.

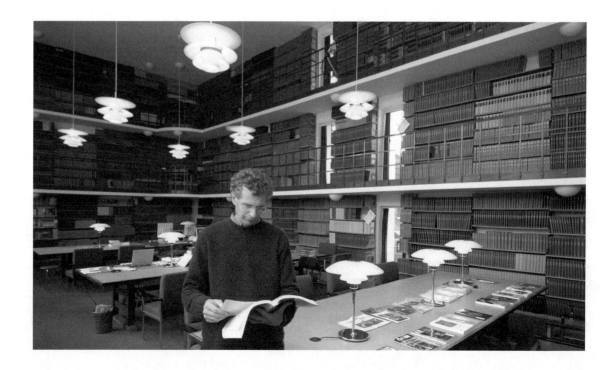

From DHGP to NGFN

In June 1995, Germany joined the international efforts of the Human Genome Project. The German Human Genome Project (Deutsches Humangenomprojekt, DHGP) was supported by the Federal Ministry of Education and Research and the Deutsche Forschungsgemeinschaft. The Resource Center located at the Max Planck Institute for Molecular Genetics, Berlin, and at the German Cancer Research Center is the central service unit. It generates, collects and administers standardized reference material and provides its services to research groups of the DHGP and also to other scientists.

Since 2001, the Ministry of Education and Research has supported the National Genome Research Network. Its aim is to explore the role that genes play in various diseases and, on this basis, to develop appropriate methods of diagnosis and treatment.

The NGFN is structured in five disease-related "Genome Networks" focusing on the study of common diseases (cancer, cardiovascular diseases, infection and inflammation, diseases of the nervous system, diseases due to environmental factors). The Cancer Network "Systems Biology of Embryonal Tumors – Neuroblastoma as a Model" is coordinated by Professor Manfred Schwab from the DKFZ; Professor Otmar D. Wiestler, DKFZ's Scientific Director, coordinates the Brain Tumor Network.

Twelve so-called Systematic Methodological Platforms (SMPs) are operating parallel to the Genome Networks. The SMPs apply and refine technologies such as high-throughput analysis or data utilization. Scientists from the DKFZ are coordinators of the SMPs "Epigenetics" (Dr. Jörg Hoheisel), "RNA" (Prof. Annemarie Poustka), "Cell" (PD Dr. Stefan Wiemann) and "Bioinformatics" (Prof. Roland Eils).

In 18 "Explorative Projects", the NGFN supports new technologies that are not yet ready for immediate application. Two such projects at the DKFZ are headed by PD Dr. Ursula Klingmüller and Dr. Ralf Bischoff.

"All these are pretty much routine tests, if you're investigating five or ten proteins", says Stefan Wiemann. "But we were thinking in dimensions of several thousand." That means that the test methods first had to be adapted to be performed automatically by liquid-handling robots – high-throughput test is the technical term. The relevance of these tests eventually depends on the statistical analysis of the data gathered in order to filter out real results. There are plans to study further parameters once the tests are ready for large-scale use.

"An isolated result in one of our functional tests is not very meaningful", says Wiemann. "More important for us is to see whether the results of different tests, together with the subcellular localization, all tell a consistent story. From the most exciting stories, we derive working hypotheses which may then be further explored at our Division of Molecular Genome Analysis."

Sibylle Kohlstädt

Literature

Mehrle, A. et al.: Nucleic Acids Res., in press, 2006
Arlt, D. et al.: Cancer Res. 65:7733, 2005
Wiemann, S. et al.: Genome Res. 14:2136, 2004

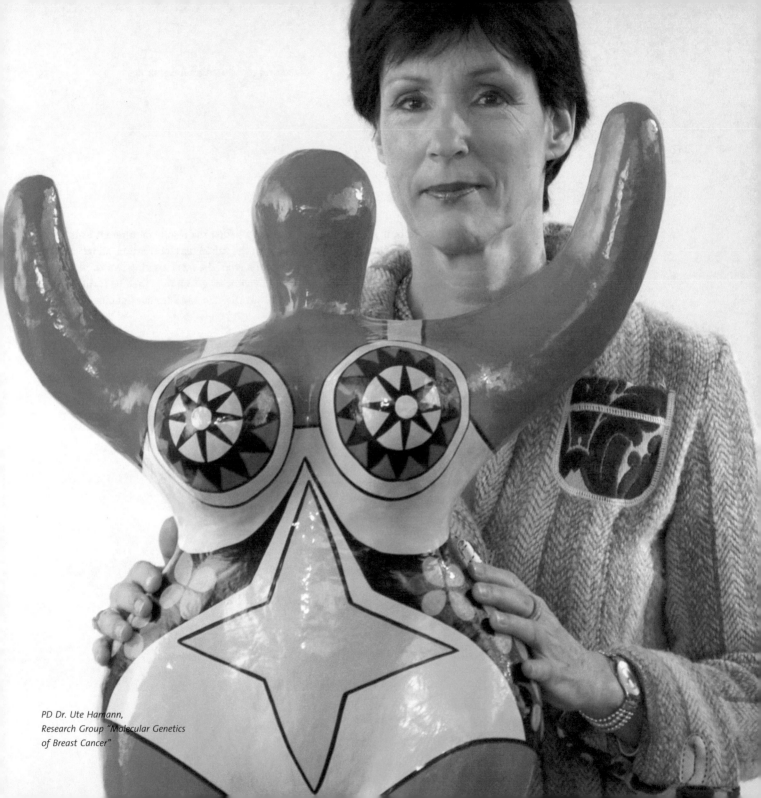

PD Dr. Ute Hamann,
Research Group "Molecular Genetics
of Breast Cancer"

Of Breast Cancer Genes and Their Accomplices

Alongside mutations in the known "breast cancer genes", BRCA1 and BRCA2, there are other genetic

variants – called polymorphisms – that influence the risk of developing breast cancer

It is a sad world record: Breast cancer is not only at the top of the list of most frequent tumors in women, it is also the second most common cancer worldwide. Moreover, breast cancer is the most frequent cause of cancer death in women. In Germany alone, about 48,000 new cases are diagnosed each year – that means that one in ten women in this country will be diagnosed with a malignant knot in her breast at some point in her life. About every third breast cancer sufferer dies of the disease. The figures are alarming. Therefore, researchers are putting a lot of effort into investigating the causes of this disease.

"We already know various genetic alterations that are associated with an elevated breast cancer risk", explains PD Dr. Ute Hamann, head of the Research Group "Molecular Genetics". She adds: "But other factors such as diet, hormone replacement therapy, hormonal contraception, age at first period and at menopause, number of children and a woman's age when she first gave birth, also seem to play a role." Nevertheless, medics and natural scientists are still unable to define the exact cause of the disease or assess individual risks – apart from a few cases of a family history of breast cancer.

A Question of Genes

A first, important step towards understanding the disease was the deciphering of the breast cancer genes BRCA1 and BRCA2. Their gene products play a role in numerous cellular processes and, as tumor suppressors, prevent uncontrolled multiplication of cells (see box on page 60). Mutations in these genes lead to a loss of the controlling function – at least, if both copies in the genetic material (called alleles) are affected.

A woman who inherits a defective BRCA allele has an increased risk of developing the hereditary form of breast and ovarian cancer. For a complete loss of function it is enough if the second gene copy gets damaged and ceases to work – e.g. under the influence of carcinogenic substances. Therefore, about 60 to 80 percent of mutation carriers are diagnosed with breast cancer at some point in their lives; ovarian cancer is

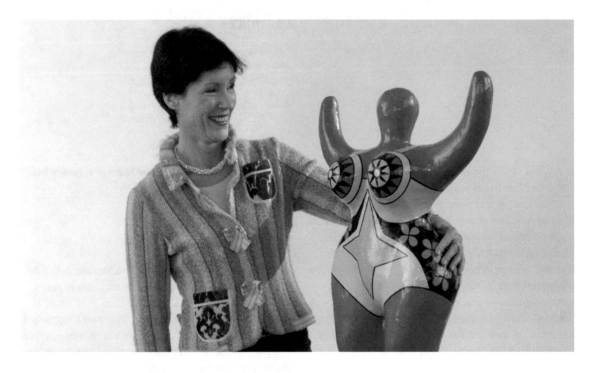

diagnosed in 15 to 40 percent of affected women. They usually develop the disease at an earlier age than women in whom the defects in both gene copies of a cell have occurred in the course of their lifetime.

However clear the role of BRCA mutations in the development of breast cancer, they explain only a very small portion of cases. It is estimated that these alterations are responsible for no more than two per-cent of breast cancers. Not even the presence of a BRCA mutation allows one to make a definite statement about the actual breast cancer risk. "Although the chance of developing breast or ovarian cancer is extremely elevated in these cases, it still does not happen to every mutation carrier", says Hamann. What is more: There are even differences in related women carrying the very same alteration in the genetic material. Some women develop tumors in the breast, others in the ovaries.

"If we want to learn more about breast cancer and its risks, we have to approach the problem from two sides", the scientist explains. "On the one hand, we need to take a close look at the different BRCA mutations, and on the other, we need to look for factors influencing the susceptibility to breast cancer." These may be environmental influences, but also further genetic characteristics that have an effect on the disease risk.

In Germany, a large variety of familial BRCA mutations are found. These are distributed across the entire gene and only few occur frequently. On the basis of this variety it is extremely difficult to determine the risks associated with each individual genetic alteration. However, things look different in other regions of the world. There are population groups in which a few, common mutations are responsible for the clustering of breast and ovarian cancer cases in some families. "What we know about common BRCA mutations is that most of these are so-called founder mutations, which often occurred hundreds of years ago and usually have been passed on within a culture or ethnic group or in a geographically limited region", explains Hamann.

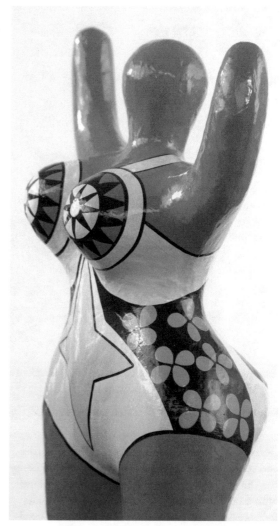

Controlling Authorities in the Genome

"Breast cancer genes" – this term, applied to the BRCA1 and BRCA2 genes, is misleading. Nature has not provided for a gene for a specific cancer in our cells. Instead, these are genes known as tumor suppressor genes, whose products eliminate DNA damage and control the cell cycle and, thus, the multiplication of cells. However, mutations in the respective parts of the genome may lead to a loss of these controlling authorities and may be the first and crucial step towards cancer development. Alterations in the arrangement of nucleic acids are known in both genes – scattered across their entire lengths. They lead to defective gene products and familial clustering of breast and ovarian cancer cases in affected families.

BRCA1 is located on the long arm of chromosome 17 and codes for a protein that is built from 1.863 amino acid building blocks and is found in a number of human tissues such as the breast, ovaries, testicles and thymus. BRCA2, located on the long arm of chromosome 13, is even larger than BRCA1 and comprises 3.418 amino acids. Similar to BRCA1, it is found in a whole number of tissues.

The products of both breast cancer genes interact with a multitude of regulatory proteins and are involved in numerous cellular processes. BRCA1 plays an important role in DNA repair, transcriptional regulation, cell cycle control, tagging of proteins to be degraded and disposed of – a process called ubiquitination –, and chromatin organization. BRCA2 is important for DNA repair and regulation of cell division.

Breast Cancer in Columbia, Pakistan and Poland

Hence, Ute Hamann's work spans different countries and continents. In Columbia, jointly with colleagues of the University of Bogotá, she is studying 60 families with a familial history of breast cancer. First results indicate a specific mutation pattern, which is a good starting basis for further investigations. Furthermore, the Heidelberg molecular biologist is involved in a study of the Shaukat Khanum Memorial Cancer Hospital in Lahore, Pakistan, which is the country with the highest incidence of breast cancer in the whole of Asia. But the high incidence rates are not the only reason why Pakistan is relevant for Hamann and colleagues.

"Another significant fact is that so many women are affected, although almost all of them give birth to several children and also rather early in their lives." This shows that two typical non-genetic risk factors for breast and ovarian cancers, namely childlessness and giving birth at a later age, do not contribute to cancer development in Pakistani patients. "The results we have obtained so far show that BRCA1 und BRCA2 are responsible for the development of a large portion of hereditary cases in Pakistan", says Hamann, summarizing what is known so far. "They also indicate that there must be further genes that are involved in the development of hereditary breast cancer. We aim to identify these in the next few years."

Within the framework of an ongoing study in Poland, Hamann has already made significant advances in this search. Working together with Polish and Australian colleagues, she is studying naturally occurring variants in genes, known as polymorphisms, which influence tumor development. These can be variants of genes whose products play a role, for example, in hormone biosynthesis or DNA repair, in signal transduction chains influencing growth, or in the metabolization of substances of endogenous or exogenous origin. The variants alone do not cause the disease. However, they can lessen or increase an existing risk such as the presence of a BRCA mutation. This is why they are referred to as risk-modifying gene variants. To know these is eminently important for early detection screenings and monitoring of women who are at a high risk of developing hereditary breast cancer.

In the Polish study subjects, researchers were able to identify two polymorphisms which additionally increase the cancer risk in BRCA1 mutation carriers. One of these gene variants is associated with a twofold increase of breast cancer risk for those carrying it – no matter which of the two commonest BRCA1 founder mutations they carry. For BRCA1 mutation carriers in whose genetic material a variant of the second identified gene was additionally found, the breast cancer risk was increased threefold.

Sporadic Breast Cancer in Germany

When there is no familial clustering, scientists speak of "sporadic" breast cancer cases, which are much more common. For these, too, scientists are trying to find out the genetic and non-genetic factors contributing to the disease. This is the aim of a German study named

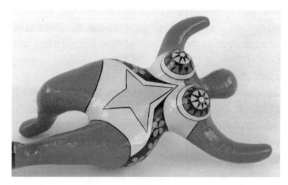

GENICA (*Gene Environment Interactions and Breast Cancer in Germany*; www.GENICA.de). Scientists from different institutes and disciplines have joined together in this large-scale project to elucidate both the environmental and the genetic causes of sporadic breast cancer.

In this study, Ute Hamann was responsible, together with her colleagues in Stuttgart, Dr. Christina Justenhoven and PD Dr. Hiltrud Brauch, for the molecular-genetic investigations. When they compared patients with healthy study participants, the scientists discovered several gene variants which they consider relevant for the development of breast cancer. One of these is ERCC2, whose product is involved both in DNA repair and in programmed cell death, or apoptosis, which is designed, among other things, to eliminate cells that are irreparably damaged. Two polymorphisms of the ERCC2 gene were particularly significant: One was found to be correlated with a twofold increase of breast cancer risk, the other with a 3.5-fold increase. In the case of CHEK2, however, the scientists did not find their assumptions confirmed. The gene product of CHEK2 acts as a guardian of genomic integrity and plays a key role in the cellular response to DNA damage. CHEK2 controls a multitude of proteins that are involved in stopping a cell's multiplication cycle, activating DNA repair, or apoptosis. Contrary to what scientists had assumed, this polymorphism is not relevant for the chance of developing sporadic breast cancer. "While a single variant has only a minor effect on cancer risk, different polymorphisms taken together can add up", says Ha-

mann, explaining the relevance of the molecular-biological results. "It is certain that the susceptibility to breast cancer both of the hereditary and the sporadic types is determined by specific sequence variants in the genetic material." In addition, the identified polymorphisms also provide clues about other mechanisms in the body which also play a role in the development of breast cancer and, thus, contribute to a better understanding of the disease.

A Closer Look at Hormone Replacement Therapy

The next project of the GENICA scientists, working together with colleagues of the MARIE working group, is to take a closer look at the relationship between hormone replacement therapy and breast cancer risk. MARIE (a German acronym that stands for "breast cancer risk factor survey") is a collaboration of researchers from the German Cancer Research Center and a number of Hamburg research institutes. When studying the influence of environmental factors and lifestyle on disease rates, scientists of the GENICA group noticed a conspicuous frequency of diagnosed breast cancers in women who had taken hormone drugs over a prolonged period of time. Previous studies in the U.S. and the U.K. had provided similar evidence. But for hormone replacement therapy, too, there are different risk groups. "It is not surprising that the female organism reacts with varying sensitivity to the hormones given", says Hamann, who will again be involved in the molecular-genetic investiga-

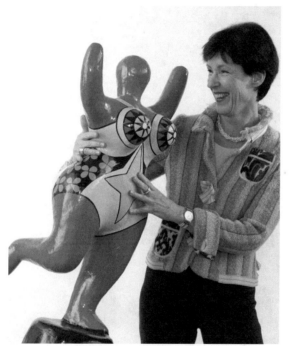

tions to be performed within this study. With a view to her future work she adds: "It is again possible that polymorphisms in hormone-associated genes play a role here – and once we have identified these, our results may influence therapy recommendations for menopausal problems. Thus, we hope to make a contribution to preventing breast cancer."

Stefanie Reinberger

Literature

Hamann, U.: BIOspektrum 10:504, 2004
Justenhoven, C. et al.: Cancer Epidemiol. Biomarker Prev. 3:2059, 2004
Rashid, M.U. et al.: Eur. J. Cancer 41:2816, 2005

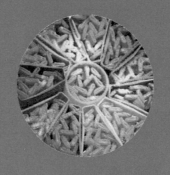

Research Program
Cancer Risk Factors and Prevention

It is a task of the Research Program to identify, quantify and determine the interactions of environmental and genetic cancer risk factors. The goal is to make a contribution to what is called primary prevention, the avoidance of cancer-causing substances or behaviors. The Research Program supports the development of early detection methods, called cancer screening measures, and tests their suitability for large population groups. In addition, working groups are searching for substances that are able to prevent progression of pre-cancerous lesions and, thus, may be used for chemoprevention. A further task of the Research Program is to search for biomarkers, i.e. characteristic molecules that can be detected in the blood or urine and allow easy and safe early detection of cancer.

Several divisions are involved in large-scale international epidemiological studies. The Biostatistics Division supports experimentally working colleagues at the Center in the design and evaluation of their studies.

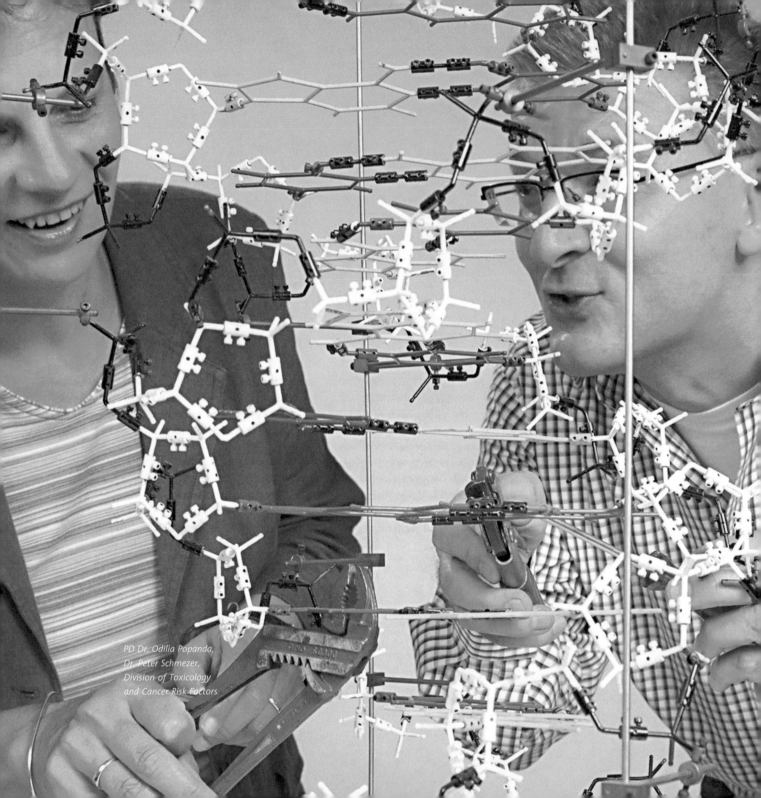

PD Dr. Odilia Popanda,
Dr. Peter Schmezer,
Division of Toxicology
and Cancer Risk Factors

Early Warning: Monitoring the Repair System

Many genes are found in a number of variants in a population. These differences in the genetic text can influence an individual's cancer risk

Everybody has an example in their families: A grand-uncle who was a chain smoker all his life and cared little about his health in general, but who lived to be as old as Methuselah without ever being seriously ill. Everybody also knows of a convinced health preacher, who avoided alcohol and cigarettes all his or her life and preferred to eat only home-grown vegetables, but who died prematurely nonetheless. This suggests that it is not only our lifestyle that determines which diseases affect us and how high our individual cancer risk is.

Professor Helmut Bartsch and his colleagues from the Division of Toxicology and Cancer Risk Factors have devoted themselves to finding out which factors play a role in tumor development. The investigation site is the human genome, because this is where changes occur that contribute to cell transformation. Thus, it is known, for example, that contact with harmful substances leaves characteristic footprints in the genetic material. Such substances or their metabolic products can attach themselves to the DNA and become what are called DNA adducts, which are responsible for er-

rors in the reading process of the genetic information. An increased number of such alterations in the genome of an individual means that his or her cancer risk is elevated.

Searching for Clues in the Genome

"We know that individuals have different risks of getting cancer due to their genetic make-up", says Bartsch's colleague, biologist Dr. Peter Schmezer. Jointly with his coworker, biochemist PD Dr. Odilia Popanda, Schmezer is investigating such genetic characteristics. An inherited elevated cancer risk can be caused, for example, by mutations, i.e. alterations in specific genes due to which a protein is not or only defectively produced. But the researchers are interested primarily in naturally occurring variations in the genome. Numerous genes occur in several different variants, called polymorphisms, in a population. These are differences in the genetic code which are hardly noticeable in healthy persons, but can have an influence on an individual's cancer risk – for example,

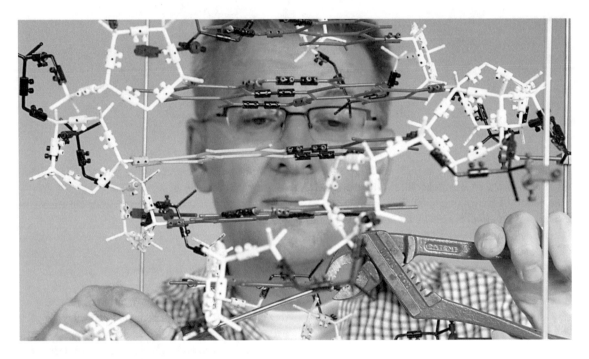

because the respective protein functions slightly better or worse. "Our goal is to identify different polymorphisms in the human genome that may serve as biomarkers for carcinogenesis und enable us to make predictions about the individual cancer risk", says Popanda, describing her research.

The two scientists and their team are focusing their search on cellular DNA repair mechanisms. These are, to a large extent, responsible for preventing that every little defect in the DNA leads to a catastrophe. Our genetic material gets damaged all the time – by environmental influences as well as aggressive products of our body's own metabolism such as reactive oxygen compounds. Usually, the body's own repair troops act quickly by spotting damaged regions, removing defective building blocks and repairing the genetic material. However, if this fails, the defective building block can lead to a copying error which is passed on when the cell divides next time. This represents a first step towards cancer development.

The devastating effects of a defective repair system become apparent, for example, in a hereditary disease called Xeroderma pigmentosum. Due to a genetic defect in those affected, altered DNA building blocks are not cut out – such as the tight bonds between adjacent thymidine bases which are considered to be typical UV light damages. The fatal result is: Every contact with sunlight leads to irreparable damages in the DNA of a sufferer's skin cells and, thus, creates more and more sites of cancer development. "It is rare that the link between carcinogenesis and defective repair mechanisms is as obvious as in this case", says Schmezer. "But still, we are sure that we are on the right track, because the elimination of constantly occurring damages is of tremendous relevance."

Scoring DNA Repair Systems

A couple of years ago, Schmezer and his colleague Popanda developed a test allowing one to make statements about the individual performance of repair enzymes. To this end, he first takes blood samples from study subjects and adds a DNA damaging substance to the white blood cells. The substance loosens up the normally densely compressed DNA and even induces breaks in some places. In a technology called single cell gel electrophoresis, a cell thus treated is then brought into an electrical field where its DNA starts migrating and, like a comet, leaves a bright tail behind – an effect that gave this test its name: Comet Assay. The crucial point is that the tail gets the longer,

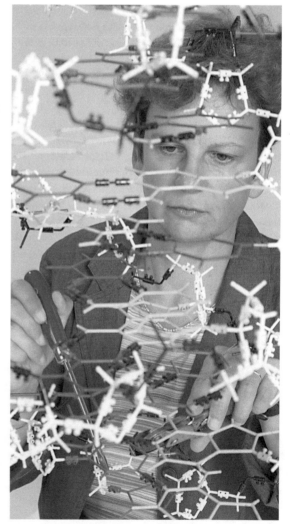

the more breaks there are, i.e., the more severely damaged the genetic material is. "In this way, we can determine how well the cell was able to repair DNA damages. The shorter the tail, the better the repair troops were able to repair the toxically induced DNA breaks", explains Popanda.

A first practical test conducted in collaboration with medics of Heidelberg Thorax Clinic has shown that the tail lengths of blood cells of persons suffering from lung cancer – non-small cell bronchial carcinoma, to be more precise – in the Comet Assay are much bigger compared to healthy study subjects. "Despite these promising results, we are still a long way from clinical application of this prognosis method", Schmezer emphasizes. Popanda adds: "In addition, the Comet Assay can only serve as a kind of rapid test, since it does not tell us which component of the repair system has failed."

To date, scientists know more than 130 enzymes that are involved in repairing DNA damages. These are able to support each other and, thus, for example, compensate a non-working member. Some of these enzymes are responsible for different damages and therefore often play a role in different types of cancer. "This is why we are not only interested in repair enzymes altogether, but also in individual members and their genetic variations", says Schmezer. He is referring, in particular, to those polymorphisms, in which only a single DNA building block (nucleotide) varies. These so-called SNPs (single nucleotide polymorphisms, pronounced "snips") occur rather frequently in our genetic material, every few thousand base pairs. A number of these are associated with a susceptibility to various diseases.

Schmezer and Popanda started looking for such tiny variations in DNA repair genes that might have an influence on lung cancer risk. To help them search, they used a technique called DNA melting point analysis

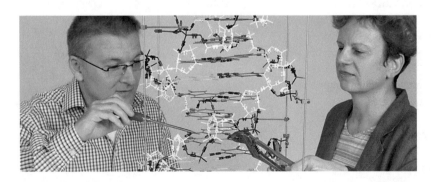

Repair enzymes correct defects in the DNA double strand

What the Melting Point Tells Us

An elegant method to identify SNPs, tiny variants in the genetic material, is called melting point analysis. To this end, the genome regions of interest are first amplified by polymerase chain reaction (PCR).

Next, the researchers need what is called a hybridization probe pair: One of these short synthetic DNA fragments is exactly complementary to the region containing the SNP, the other one to an adjacent sequence. Each probe is labeled with a different fluorescent dye. The light emitted by one dye excites the other one, which then also emits light. Thus, a measurable light signal is obtained only when both fragments have attached themselves to the target genome region. And again, only if the positions of the two probes are directly adjacent.

The melting point helps to distinguish between two possible sequence variants at the SNP location. The target DNA is melted at high temperatures into sin-gle strands and the hybridization probes are then given the opportunity to attach themselves to the DNA.

When the mixture is reheated, the hybridization probes detach themselves from the DNA and the light signal ceases. The temperature at which this happens – the melting point – is the higher, the more exactly a DNA fragment and a probe match each other. If a single building block of the probe varies from the "master copy" of genomic DNA, it will detach itself at lower temperatures than in the case of exactly complementary binding partners. Since the base sequence of the probe is known, scientists can infer the genomic sequence in the area of the SNP.

If several SNPs are to be investigated in the same gene, the melting point analysis needs to be carried out in parallel runs, each with matching hybridization probe pairs.

(see box on page 71). The scientists thus studied the genome of 463 lung cancer patients with non-small cell bronchial carcinoma and of 460 control persons. In doing so, they kept an eye on both the normal version and variations of various repair genes whose products are in charge of cutting out inappropriate or damaged building blocks or mending breaks in the DNA strand. Indeed, they found a correlation between specific SNPs and cancer risk. Thus, a variant of a gene called APE1 appears to provide better protection against cancer, while certain versions of the XPA, XPD, and XRCC3 genes were found to increase the chances of cancer. In addition, it turned out that a combination of several high-risk variations additionally increases the risk of getting cancer. "These conspicuous variants may one day serve as biomarkers to determine the lung cancer risk", says Popanda. "But we need to emphasize time and again that we are still a long way from a testing method for use in clinical practice."

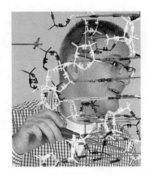

DNA repair mechanisms also become active in case of radiation damage

Helping to Make Treatment Decisions

With their most recent project, the two researcher are leaving the area of prognosis and prevention in order to investigate the relevance of polymorphisms on the results of radiotherapy. "Radiation, even if focused with the utmost precision on the tumor, not only destroys cancer cells, but can also damage healthy cells", says Schmezer. In sensitive patients, this can manifest itself in inflammations and poorly healing wounds,

which, in serious cases, can lead to a loss of tissue function. In this case, radiation therapy has to be terminated before it has achieved its actual goal of tumor destruction.

Radiation damage is another case where cellular DNA repair mechanisms become active and are responsible for an individual patient's susceptibility. Again, Popanda and Schmezer suspected an influence of the small gene variations and started working with medics and epidemiologists in Heidelberg, Mannheim and Karlsruhe to look for polymorphisms. This investigation was focused on breast cancer patients receiving radiation therapy. Again, in a number of repair genes that are responsible for cutting out inappropriate DNA regions, SNPs were identified which are related to a particular radiation susceptibility. Particularly interesting were variants of the APE1 gene known already from lung cancer as well as polymorphisms in the

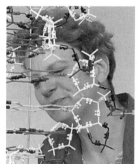

Specific polymorphisms in the genes of repair enzymes make a cell particularly radiation-sensitive

The benefit of such biomarkers for the choice of treatment is apparent. But what could be the advice to a person whose cancer risk has been determined? Would he or she be given a "license" to smoke, for example, just because his or her repair mechanisms are working better? "By no means", emphasizes Schmezer. "If our markers will eventually be applied in clinical practice, they will only provide information about the work of the repair systems, but this does not tell us anything about other genetically determined factors." It is more likely that persons with a particularly high risk, which may also have manifested itself in various cancer cases in the family, may be given the advice to have regular prevention exams so as to detect tumors early and increase the chances of cure.

Stefanie Reinberger

Literature

Schmezer, P. et al.: Mutagenesis 16:25, 2001

Popanda, O. et al.: Carcinogenesis 25:2433, 2004

Bartsch, H. et al.: Spektrum der Wissenschaft Spezial: Krebsmedizin II, Seite 46, 2003

XRCC1 gene. "By identifying such SNPs we are hoping to one day provide physicians with a tool that helps them in deciding whether and what dose of radiation therapy is suitable for a patient", Popanda summarizes the results of this investigation. Doctors are also hoping that such SNPs might be suitable biomarkers to assess possible delayed effects of radiotherapy.

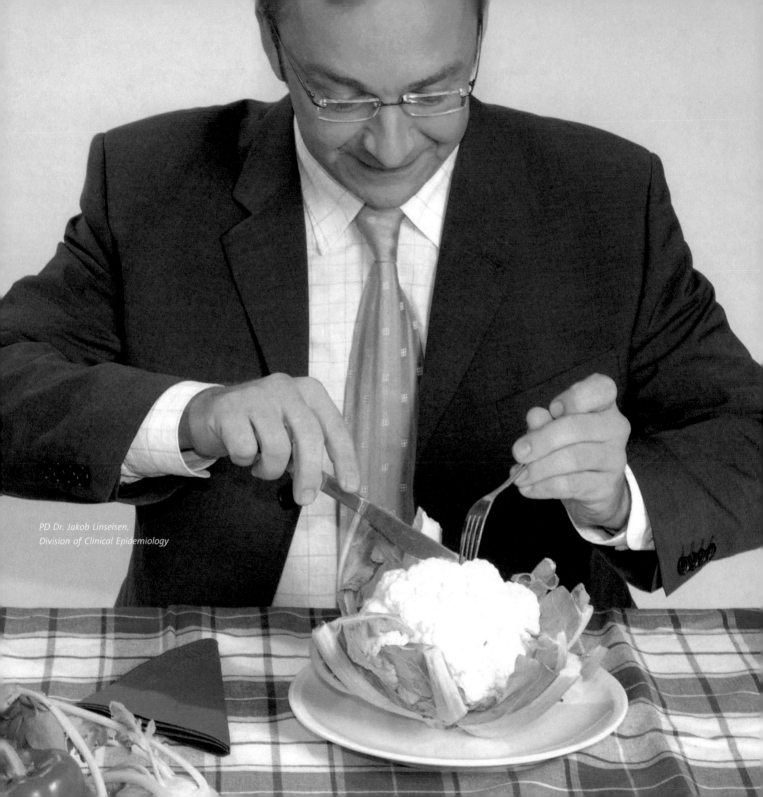

PD Dr. Jakob Linseisen,
Division of Clinical Epidemiology

A Question of Diet

Scientists throughout Europe are conducting the EPIC study in the hope that cancer prevention will enter every household through the grocery list

Scientists today attribute a remarkably large proportion of cancer cases – about 35 percent – to dietary factors. As a risk factor, nutrition thus carries the same weight as smoking, but it is much more complicated to assess. While we can identify cigarettes or alcohol as single influence factors, it is much more difficult to pin down the effects of a myriad of foodstuffs and their components, along with their manifold combination possibilities.

To take a closer look at the links between specific dietary habits and cancer, a Europe-wide study was initiated: "EPIC" is devoted to studying the connections between dietary factors and cancer and other chronic diseases. Since 1992, more than 520,000 Europeans in ten countries have served cancer research by having their body measurements and blood samples taken and completing questionnaires about their dietary habits and lifestyles. In addition, they have agreed to be available for data updates every two years. The aim is to obtain possibly detailed information about the grocery lists of Europeans and resulting cancer risks (see box on page 77).

Scientists are aware that it will be a long time before they can reap results. Before any reliable statistical conclusions can be drawn, a sufficient number of cases is needed. This is the reason why results for common cancers such as tumors of the colon and rectum, breast, prostate, and lung are expected to be reached first. Scientists will have to accept this time factor, whether they like it or not. For only a study of this type, called a prospective study, in which information and blood samples are collected before a possible diagnosis, ensures the required accuracy. If persons already afflicted were questioned about their prior dietary habits, their memory and, thus, the results of the survey would be distorted by their knowledge of being diagnosed with the disease.

Please Help Yourselves: Fruits, Vegetables and Fish

What are the findings of EPIC roughly one decade after it started? Scientists have indeed been able to start evaluations for the most common cancers and have published the first meaningful data. Thus, under the leadership of the Heidelberg EPIC team, then headed by Professor Antony B. Miller, a proven connection between lung cancer and the intake of fruits was established: The more fruits study subjects ate, the lower was their risk to develop cancer of the respiratory tract. The connection was particularly apparent in smokers. They were the only group in which vegetables – alongside fruits – also helped to lower the risk of lung cancer.

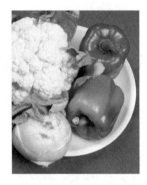

EPIC has shown: Fruits and vegetables have no influence on breast cancer risk

However, what applies to the lung is not automatically transferable to other organs. An investigation on breast cancer, for example, suggested no connection between disease risk and the regular intake of vegetables and fruits. EPIC investigators have thus confuted the results of case-control studies with breast cancer patients where the evaluation suggested such a connection. "As to breast cancer, factors influencing a woman's hormone situation play a primary role, such as the number of births, duration of breastfeeding, whether she had hormone therapy and age at menopause", says PD Dr. Jakob Linseisen, who has led the Heidelberg EPIC team since May 2004. Results obtained by the Heidelberg researchers suggest that the latter also seems to be influenced by dietary factors.

Another organ that has been the object of scrutiny so far is the bowel (colon and rectum). Since EPIC started, 1,329 cases of colorectal cancer were diagnosed among study participants. A recent evaluation of 2005 has shown a link between the intake of meat and sausage products and the risk of this type of tumor. Study subjects who frequently consume what is called "red" (muscle) meat such as pork, beef or lamb were afflicted more often than participants whose menu only rarely includes these foods. Epidemiologists estimate that the risk of colorectal cancer increases by 50% per 100 grams of daily consumed red meat. Things are even worse for sausage products, which increase the risk by 70%. A possible explanation offered by epidemiologists is that the iron taken in with the meat may lead to the formation of harmful nitroso compounds in the bowel. This could also be the reason why regular consumption of poultry has no influence on colorectal cancer incidence. The meat of chicken & Co contains much less iron than that of the mammals which usually end up on our plates. The mode of preparation, such as searing and conservation methods such as salting and smoking, might also play a role.

Half a Million Europeans in the Service of Cancer Research

For some twelve years now, 520,000 Europeans have been serving the cause of science. At regular intervals – approximately every two years – they answer questions about their dietary habits and health status. Thus, they contribute to a the EPIC project (European Prospective Investigation into Cancer and Nutrition), the largest ever European study investigating the role of diet and lifestyle, metabolism, and genetic factors in the development of cancer and other chronic diseases.

Although there are similar studies in the United States, lifestyle and dietary habits on the two continents are too different to allow a simple transfer of results from the New World to the Old World. Thus, on the other side of the Atlantic ocean, food additives play a more important role than here. Another argument in favor of a separate European study is that it involves a huge body of participants covering an enormous range of different lifestyles and diets.

EPIC was started in 1992 under the coordination of Dr. Elio Riboli at the International Agency for Research on Cancer (IARC) in Lyon, France (since 11/05 Imperial College, London). Since then scientists from originally seven different nations – Germany, France, Greece, the United Kingdom, Italy, the Netherlands,

and Spain – have been collecting data in the populations of their respective countries. The Scandinavian countries, Denmark, Norway and Sweden, had already been involved in a similar study and joined the project soon after. All information gathered by the participating institutes is centrally pooled and subsequently evaluated by various research groups.

Two study centers are located in Germany: at the German Institute of Human Nutrition (Deutsches Institut für Ernährungsforschung, DIfE) in Potsdam and the German Cancer Research Center (Deutsches Krebsforschungszentrum, DKFZ) in Heidelberg. The Heidelberg researchers started collecting data in 1994 and were able to recruit more than 25,500 volunteers from Heidelberg and the surrounding area. The study participants between the ages of 35 and 65 years – 53 percent of which are women and 47 percent are men – completed questionnaires and were additionally interviewed about various aspects of their dietary and living habits. The blood samples provided by almost all participants are stored in liquid nitrogen. These are used for measuring suitable indicators, called biomarkers, for food intake, metabolism and hereditary susceptibility – and, thereby, also for evaluating the interplay of all these factors in the sense of gene-environment interactions. Furthermore, the amount of time that has passed between taking the blood and cancer diagnosis is known for each blood sample. This is why the EPIC sample collections are ideal for testing tumor markers for their suitability for early detection.

From the beginning, the Heidelberg study participants have been asked regularly by mail to report on newly diagnosed diseases and changes in the exposure factors – both dietary and environmental. German scientists are struggling with a special problem here: There is no functioning nationwide cancer register in this country. Therefore, epidemiologists in Germany have to request information from doctor's offices and hospitals to collect additional data which in other countries have long since been kept in central registers. Thus, the success of the EPIC study depends most of all on the continuing willingness of study subjects to provide information.

In contrast, regular consumption of fish protects against cancer of the colon and/or rectum. According to the same evaluation, 100 grams more fish daily reduce the risk of colorectal cancer by one half. Scientists assume that this may be caused by the high content of omega-3 fatty acids. These fatty acids influence the production of tissue hormones and also have anti-inflammatory effects.

A discussion that has been going on for many years is whether dietary fiber protects against bowel cancer. This question has also been addressed by EPIC investigators. A first evaluation of 2003 had already shown that a high-fiber diet has a protective effect on the bowel. A more recent publication confirms this finding: In the group with the highest intake of dietary fiber the risk of colorectal cancer was reduced by up to 40 percent – at least with respect to the left half of the colon. For this effect it did not seem to matter whether the dietary fiber came from whole grains, vegetables, or fruits.

Refining the Measurement Methods

Critics of the European large-scale study may argue that EPIC study participants might rationalize their lifestyle by stating that they consume much more fruits and vegetables or less alcohol than they really do. Jakob Linseisen rebuts this criticism: "Of course we have to allow for some inaccuracy in our survey", the epidemiologist concedes, "but we have taken account of this as best we can in the design of the study and the evaluations." Thus, in the scientific evaluations study subjects are not evaluated by absolute amounts of specific foods, but by groups, for example, whether they eat no fruits at all or only little or even a lot of it. This alone will even out many imprecise statements.

"Additionally, we work with what we call 24-hour re-calls in which subjects have to state what they ate the day before", Linseisen explains. Since it is not diffi-cult to recall yesterday's menu, the investigators ob-tain very exact data in these additional surveys. These can be used to "calibrate" the other results. This meth-od is employed for the first time ever in a study of this kind. In EPIC, it is also used to even out country-specific differences in the diet questionnaires: While,

for example, subjects from Norway answer more ques-tions relating to fish intake, German study partici-pants are asked more questions about their bread con-sumption – tailored to country-specific preferences. The 24-hour recalls, however, are the same for all par-ticipants and, thus, allow to make precise statements about dietary habits at the individual EPIC centers. Another independent measure for nutrient supply that is available to the scientists are the collected blood samples that allow to identify nutrients such as folic acid, carotinoids, or vitamin C.

No End in Sight

Relevant as these first results of the EPIC study are, they are but small puzzle pieces. The road to a com-plete picture is still long. Therefore, epidemiologists will continue to collect data over the next few years so that they will also be able, step by step, to make statements about rarer cancers. For some cancers, such as lymphomas and brain tumors, oncologists have only little knowledge about influenceable risk factors so far. Moreover, genetic components such as poly-morphisms, i.e. tiny variations in the genetic material found in populations, will play a role in future evalua-tions. For epidemiologists are asking themselves whether certain dietary factors might have a different influence in persons with a genetically determined predisposition for a disease than in persons without this characteristic.

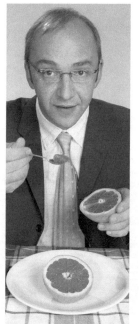

It is not yet known which components of fruits cause their protective effect against lung cancer

"But in the next few years we will also have to look more closely", Linseisen describes further goals. "Thus, instead of talking simply about lung cancer, we should start distinguishing between different forms of the disease." Tumors that differ so widely in their histology, i.e. in the way the tumor tissue looks, as small cell and non-small cell bronchial carcinomas are very likely to have different causes. As a result, it seems appropriate to look for risk factors for each type separately.

Looking more closely also means to differentiate the other side, i.e. nutrition, more accurately. "We are still talking about fruits or meat as a sort of collective term", the Heidelberg scientist explains. However, he believes that things will become much more interesting once we will be able to determine the effects of individual dietary components and their combinations. Linseisen provides an example: "In our lung cancer study, we can only speculate about which fruit components provide the protective effect. In particu-

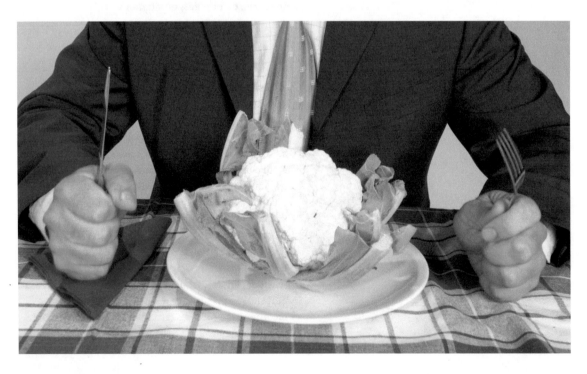

lar, studying the effects of secondary plant compounds on human health still poses many problems."

What else does Linseisen hope for the future of the study? "Certainly that we will be able to undermine and expand our knowledge with possibly unambiguous results in order to further specify current recommendations for disease prevention", the epidemiologist replies. He hesitates shortly before he continues: "To specify may also mean to issue dietary recommen-

dations based on special genetic and metabolic characteristics. But that is still a vision of the future."

Stefanie Reinberger

Literature

Bingham, S., Riboli, E.: Nat Rev Cancer 4:206, 2004
Norat, T. et al.: J Natl Cancer Inst 97:906, 2005
Miller, A. B. et al.: Int J Cancer 108:269, 2004

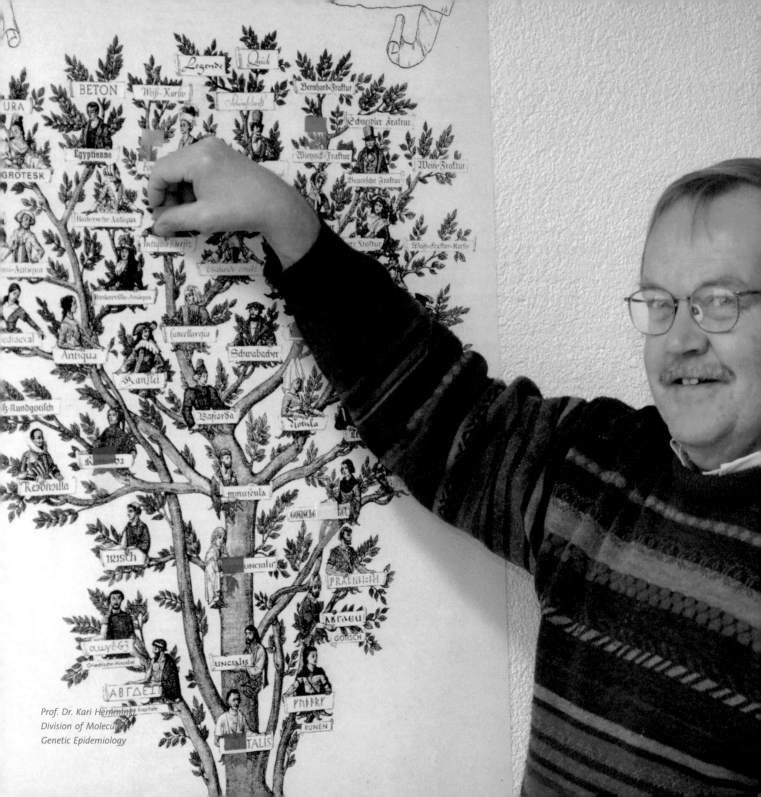

Prof. Dr. Kari Hemminki,
Division of Molecular
Genetic Epidemiology

Ancestors and other Risk Factors

In many common cancers, direct relatives of sufferers have an increased risk of developing the same type of cancer

"Cancer is a disease of the genes." This is how scientists like to summarize the complex process of how malignant tumors develop. But the sentence has already caused a great deal of confusion. Does that mean that cancer is a hereditary disease? Yes and no. Most genetic changes that are responsible for the loss of control in cell division or invasive growth happen in the course of a lifetime in a single cell of our body and are not inherited from the parents. In some families, however, the situation is different. It has been known for a long time now that inherited genetic defects play a role in cancers of the colon, breast or ovaries. In the case of inherited cancer syndromes such as the rare familial adenomatous polyposis (FAP) and the non-polyposis colorectal cancer syndrome, mutation carriers are at high risk to develop colorectal cancer before age 40. These two hereditary diseases account for roughly five to ten percent of colorectal cancer cases. Familial clustering of breast and ovarian cancers, however, are often caused by inherited mutations in the BRCA1 and BRCA2 genes (see box on page 60).

"FAP, HNPCC or BRCA – these are known mutations in high-risk genes that are highly likely to cause cancer", explains Professor Kari Hemminki, who leads the Division of Molecular Genetic Epidemiology at the DKFZ. "Apart from these, we suspect there are numerous other inherited genetic alterations that also contribute to the development of individual types of cancer, although with lower probabilities." Hemminki has good reasons for his suspicion. Working at the Karolinska Institute in Stockholm, the Finland-born researcher integrated two data collections, thus creating a unique possibility of identifying familial clusterings of cancer. To this end, he combined the Swedish Family Register, a record of all individuals born in Sweden after 1932, with the Swedish Cancer Register, which records almost 100 percent of cancer cases occurring in the population. The result was a nationwide "Family Cancer Register". By integrating both databases Hemminki and his coworkers have been able to analyze the distribution of 1.1 million cancer cases in 10.2 million people from over three million families. "The world's largest family database", says Hemminki with satisfaction.

Together with his coworkers, Dr. Xinjun Li and Dr. Kamila Czene, he set about investigating the familial distribution of the 25 most common cancers in Sweden. The researchers were somewhat surprised to find that in 24 out of 25 cancer locations under investigation, first-degree relatives (siblings or offspring) of cancer sufferers have an increased risk of getting the same cancer.

In top position, with roughly 15 percent of all familial cancer cases, is prostate cancer. Earlier studies already indicated a hereditary component in this disease, but no genes have yet been identified that play a role in the disease process. Next are colorectal cancer with 10 percent of familial cases and breast cancer with 8.5 percent of familial cases. Other cancer types such as cancers of the kidney, skin, stomach or lung can also occur in a familial form and do so more often than previously thought. Familial forms were least frequent in testicular cancer (0.5 percent) and connective tissue tumors (0.4

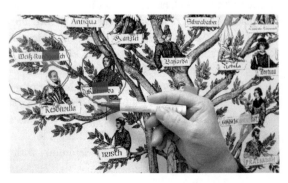

percent). Disease risks are usually particularly high if two first-degree relatives (parent and siblings) were affected by the same cancer and if they were diagnosed with this cancer at a relatively young age.

More Meaningful Information Through Absolute Numbers

The epidemiologists were not only interested in finding out which cancer types have a hereditary component, but also wanted to determine, for each cancer location, the risks of members of affected families to get the same cancer. To this end, they separately calculated the risks of offspring and of siblings of cancer sufferers. Clearly the strongest effects were found in testicular cancer: The brothers of affected individuals have a ninefold increased risk to develop this cancer compared to non-affected families. The sons of affected fathers still have a fourfold increased risk. High degrees of heritability were also determined for Hodgkin's lymphoma (risk increased 5.9 fold), kidney cancer (4.7 fold), prostate (4.5) and ovarian (4.3) cancers. However, Hemminki emphasizes that these numbers mean relative risks. "A twofold increased risk of breast cancer means for the Swedish population, on which, after all, the investigation is based, that we have to expect about 900 additional cases within a ten-year period. For a rare disease such as Hodgkin's lymphoma, a relative risk of four means no more than six additional cases in the same period."

Therefore, it is often more meaningful to express disease risks in absolute numbers. Thus, persons with a parent suffering from breast cancer have a risk of 5.5 percent to develop the same type of cancer by age 68 – compared to 3.4 percent for persons whose parents are not affected by this disease. Sons of fathers who have prostate cancer have a risk of 4.4 percent of also developing a malignant tumor of the prostate. By comparison, the risk for sons of non-affected fathers is only half as high.

Shared Environment vs. Shared Genes

Now, isn't it possible that a family history of certain cancers is caused not by genetic factors but by environmental factors shared equally by all family members? To answer this question, Hemminki compared the disease risks of married couples. These do not share the same genes but are usually exposed to the same environmental influences. Extensive sunbathing during summer vacations or a family room that is permanently full of smoke are obvious causes for increased skin or lung cancer rates in the family. However, the epidemiologists found increased risks for spouses of sufferers only in those cancers that are caused by already known and established risk factors such as tobacco smoke, sunburns or – in the case of genital cancers – human papillomaviruses. Thus, for the remaining types of cancer, increased familial risks appear to be related to genetic influences.

"This is not covered by genetic counseling", says Hemminki, complaining about the current situation. Thus, for familial forms of breast and ovarian cancer there are guidelines to decide whether a woman should be advised to be tested for mutations of BRCA1 and BRCA2. Such guidelines have recently been produced for colon cancer, too. However, considering Hemminki's results, genetic counseling should be considered for many more cancer types. Apart from the medical

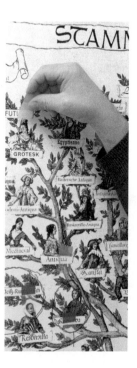

The Swedish "Family Cancer Register" documents cancer cases over several generations

Hereditary or Random?

Many women with a family history of breast and/or ovarian cancer are afraid of having a hereditary predisposition for these cancers in their genes. About five percent of all breast cancers are caused by genetic predisposition. Within the project, "Familial Breast and Ovarian Cancers", the German Cancer Aid (Deutsche Krebshilfe) supports twelve counseling centers in Germany, including one in Heidelberg, where family members of affected families can have their personal risks determined.

When a woman seeks genetic counseling, geneticists will first generate a family tree covering three generations which shows all cancer cases that have occurred among relatives. Specific criteria will then be applied to determine whether the advice-seeker does in fact belong to a family with a high genetic risk or whether it is a random increased cancer occurrence. Key indicators for genetic predisposition are breast and/or ovarian cancers in several first-degree relatives (mothers, sisters, or daughters) and early age at onset. More than one tumor in a patient as well as breast cancer in a male relative are other indicators of a familial predisposition.

If a family is classified as high-risk, it is possible to test for mutations in the BRCA1 and BRCA2 genes. If a mutation is already known in the family, then relatives can have a test to determine whether they have inherited this gene defect and, thus, a significantly higher risk to develop breast cancer or ovarian cancer. A woman carrying a BRCA1 mutation has a lifetime risk of up to 80 percent to get breast cancer. The gene test will be part of an interdisciplinary counseling concept which includes genetic and gynecological counseling and at least one psychotherapeutic session. If an advice-seeker has inherited the BRCA mutation, she will be educated about options available to her, ranging from close surveillance to preventive surgery. However, if geneticists do not detect a BRCA defect, a woman belonging to a high-risk family has no higher risk of breast or ovarian cancer than other women in the population.

For more information: www.klinikum.uni-heidelberg.de/humangenetik (Patientenversorgung, Schwerpunktprogramm Familiärer Brust- und Eierstockkrebs) or the Internet pamphlet of the Deutsche Krebshilfe: www.krebshilfe.de/neu/Infoangebot/fam_brustzentren.pdf

benefits – such as early detection through close monitoring –, this could also give affected families a sense of security.

Hemminki is certain that the Swedish Family Cancer Register will continue to be a valuable source of data for many other questions of cancer epidemiology. The high case numbers available make visible even the smallest effects, which would go unnoticed in smaller-scale investigations. Thus, the researchers are currently determining the effect of newly introduced early detection methods on the disease rate of close relatives. Using the Swedish data, they recently also calculated the percentage of cancer cases that are accounted for by individual known mutations. Thus, Hemminki's team studied families with a family his-

tory of cancer who, according to the German counseling guidelines, would be advised to be tested for mutations to breast cancer genes BRCA1 and BRCA2. Here, the epidemiologists found out that most cases of ovarian cancer, and also of other malignant tumors, were not related to BRCA mutations at all, but must be caused by other genetic alterations. To avoid that the all-clear is given too early, this is a vital piece of information for human geneticists using gene testing to assess the personal risks of members of high-risk families.

Sibylle Kohlstädt

Literature

Lorenzo Bermejo, J., Hemminki, K.: Annals of Oncology 15:1834, 2004
Hemminki, K. et al.: Int J Cancer 108:109, 2004
Hemminki, K., Eng, C.: J Med Genet 41:801, 2004

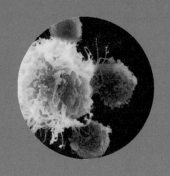

Research Program Tumor Immunology

The immune system is our body's most powerful weapon to combat pathogens and cancer cells. However, tumor cells have numerous tricks to escape the immune response. The divisions of the Research Program Tumor Immunology investigate the mechanisms regulating the behavior of immune cells. Research work focuses on cell proliferation and programmed cell death (apoptosis) as well as on the activation and regulation of immune cells. Also under investigation are cancers affecting the immune system as such. The aim is to better understand the role of the immune system in cancer, AIDS, and autoimmune diseases. The results of this research provide the basis for clinical approaches in tumor diagnosis and treatment, including the development of antibody and cell therapies, innovative vaccination strategies and tumor-specific antibodies for diagnostics.

Further working areas of the Research Program include the investigation of the connection between natural (innate) and adaptive (acquired) immunity, the investigation of the role of regulatory T cells as well as of treatment resistance of tumors, which is often caused by resistance to apoptosis-inducing signals.

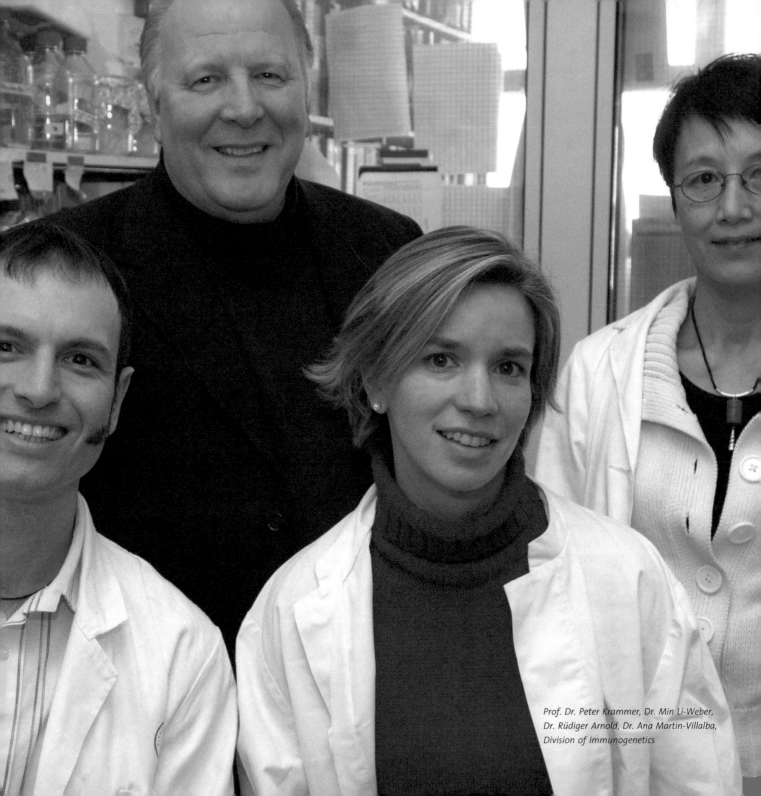

Prof. Dr. Peter Krammer, Dr. Min Li-Weber,
Dr. Rüdiger Arnold, Dr. Ana Martin-Villalba,
Division of Immunogenetics

Trademark "Apoptosis"

Apoptosis research with many facets: How is programmed cell death regulated in the immune and nervous systems? How do plant substances interfere with the complex regulation of apoptosis?

Ever since the discovery of the CD95 death receptor and the elucidation of the complex signaling cascade leading to programmed cell death, apoptosis research has been a special focus and "trademark" of the German Cancer Research Center. A name that is inseparably connected with apoptosis research is that of Peter Krammer.

When, back in the late 1980s, Peter Krammer discovered how the death cascade is triggered, nobody anticipated the key significance of apoptosis for life and death of every organism. It was not known yet that in many disease processes too much or too little apoptosis is crucial for healing or death. Today, Krammer's findings are fundamentals of cell biology, some of them have already been included in the school curricula.

When the molecular switches (see box on page 94) were discovered that cause death – also of cancer cells –, oncologists were hoping to use these mechanisms for killing tumors the "natural" way. Thus, research on apoptosis concentrated at first on its thera-

peutic use in cancer treatment. But the key role of the death program for the functioning of every organism gives rise to a much broader range of questions, especially in Krammer's own Division of Immunogenetics.

A Matter of Nerves

Medical researcher Ana Martin-Villalba focuses not on death, but on survival. She is attempting to protect cells of the central nervous system (CNS) from programmed cells death. Martin-Villalba discovered that many of the disastrous consequences of CNS traumas are caused by apoptosis. Biological processes that are happening alongside the actual trauma cause further damage to the tissue and, thus, destroy the nerve cells' ability to regenerate. In spinal cord injuries, apoptosis causes the death of nerve cells and also of oligodendrocytes – cells that produce myelin to insulate the neurons. Without myelin, neurons lose their ability to transmit signals. A similar tragedy occurs after a stroke in the brain: Here, too, cells that do not die directly for lack of oxygen, are forced to commit suicide by apoptosis. Extensive defects in the brain are the result.

Thus, Martin-Villalba's strategy was to block apoptosis in the central nervous system in order to reduce the damage caused by infarction and spinal cord injury. In experiments with mice, this therapeutic approach provided positive results in both cases. By constricting a key blood vessel in the animals' brain, the scientist caused an artificial stroke. If the animals are simulta- neously given an antibody which blocks the CD95-L protein that triggers apoptosis, the extent of tissue damage in the brain remains limited and hardly any paralysis occurred afterwards. The symptoms of a sur- gically induced paralysis also improve rapidly when the animals are injected the CD95-L antibody during spinal cord sectioning.

While both CD95-L and the death receptor protein, CD95, are found in sufficient amounts on cells of a de-

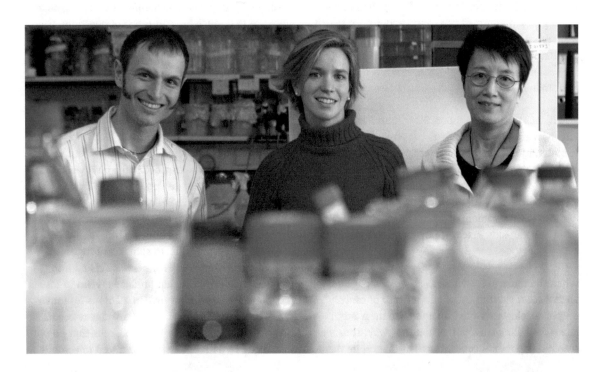

veloping brain, they are hardly detectable at a later time. This suggests that these two proteins have functions specific to development. And indeed, as shown by Martin-Villalba's most recent research, activation of CD95 in neurons of the central nervous system does not end in cell death. Quite the reverse: The scientist discovered that the nerve cells of mouse embryos that lack either CD95 or CD95-L due to a mutation form less of the branch-like protrusions called neurites, while nerves under the influence of CD95-L grow more of these cellular extensions.

Apparently, the function of the CD95 system in the developing brain is not cell death, but a growth-promoting, structure-building process. The number of neurites by which a nerve cells establishes contact with its neighbors is a measure of brain complexity. In addition, repair and regeneration processes in the CNS also rely on the sprouting of these extensions.

For Martin-Villalba, the findings suggest that the CD95 system may also play a role in regeneration processes in the adult brain. Traumas and diseases cause the death receptor and ligand levels in the brain to increase dramatically – possibly to initiate healing processes. The scientist suspects that after a trauma the presence of various messenger substances and tissue hormones at the injury site may determine whether CD95 takes the road to apoptosis or to regeneration. Martin-Villalba expects that the young neurons that develop from pluripotent cells may mature into functioning nerve cells in the presence of CD95-L. The Spanish-born scientist is determined to elucidate this balance of regeneration-promoting and -inhibiting factors in order to specifically direct nerve cells towards healing.

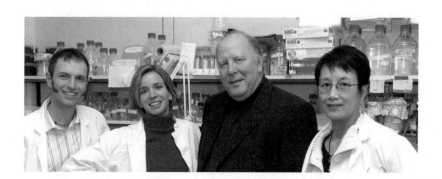

The questions may differ, but apoptosis is always the focus of research work in Peter Krammer's division

Chronicle of an Announced Death

It all began with an antibody. To study surface molecules of leukemia cells, Peter Krammer and his co-workers had produced a number of monoclonal antibodies in 1989. One of these turned out to be a real killer molecule, since it literally killed lymphocytes and various leukemia cells in the culture dish. To be more precise: The antibody triggered apoptosis, or programmed cell death. Krammer discovered that the target molecule of the killer antibody works like a switch that starts apoptosis. Soon after, researchers in his lab were able to identify the death receptor. Originally coined APO-1, it has become widely known as CD95. CD95 belongs to a group of transmembrane receptors that are related to the TNF (tumor necrosis factor) receptor. Cell death is induced when CD95, which is found on the cells of most tissues, is activated by its partner, CD95 ligand (CD95-L).

Over the following years, Krammer's team elucidated the mechanism that leads to cell death when these two molecules come into contact. On binding of CD95L, three CD95 molecules cluster with their cytoplasmatic parts called death domains. Within seconds, a complex of proteins known as "death inducing signaling complex" (DISC) is formed: The FADD adapter protein associates with the death domains. FADD, in turn, serves as a docking site for pro-caspase 8, which was originally termed FLICE by Krammer's team. Autocatalytic cleavage of pro-caspase 8 produces active caspase 8, which leaves the DISC and, by activating further caspases, initiates the final process of apoptosis.

Peter Krammer elucidated not only the complex signaling cascade that ends in the self-dissolution of the cell, but also the regulatory functions of apoptosis in immune response and viral infections. He discovered that T cells commit suicide to slow down an immune response by releasing CD95 like a messenger substance and, thus, inducing their own cell death via CD95-L-induced apoptosis. In HIV infections, the tat protein of the AIDS virus increases the amount of CD95 on T cells, which contributes to the dramatic loss of T helper cells as the disease progresses. Jointly with colleagues in Lausanne, France, Krammer found out that some viruses express inhibitors of pro-caspase 8 (FLICE) called FLIPS, which protect virus-infected cells from apoptotic elimination.

Krammer's former coworker, Dr. Henning Walczak, who leads the young scientists' group "Apoptosis Regulation" at the DKFZ today, has been focusing on a protein with promising properties: TRAIL is another member of the group of molecules that bind to death receptors of the TNF family. By binding to the TRAIL receptor, TRAIL triggers the death of tumor cells. Walczak discovered something special about this protein: Unlike CD95-L or TNF, which cause damage to all kinds of tissue in the body (e.g., systemic administration of CD95-L causes liver failure in mice), TRAIL is believed to cause no toxic side effects in mice.

A Decision on Life or Death

It was the study of our body's own defense system that put Peter Krammer on the track of programmed cell death in the late 1980s. The role of apoptosis in the process of an immune response continues to be one of the major research areas of his division. Here, scientists are currently trying to solve a question that is anything but simple: How does an immune response end?

During their development, T cells – key players in an immune response – are repeatedly forced to decide between life and death. They have to learn how to distinguish reliably between "foreign" and "self". If a cell fails at one of the steps of this quality control process, death through apoptosis is the result. If the T cell passes the test and is activated by a specific antigen that fits into the lock of the T cell receptor like a key, cell division – or clonal expansion – is the next stage. Thereby, the body ensures that the invader – virus, bacterium, or tumor cell – is encountered by a sufficiently large army of specific T cells.

However, an organism is exposed to infectious agents thousands of times during its lifetime. Each exposure triggers an expansion of T cells. To prevent that the number of immune cells grows too vast, a balance mechanism is required that both ensures a constant cell number and prevents possible attacks of misguided activated immune cells against the body's own structures. The organism achieves this by sensitizing activated T cells after the initial antigen exposure to CD95-mediated apoptosis. A process known as activation induced cell death (AICD) then reduces the number of cells to the original level.

But how does a T cell that is resistant to any death signals during the defense stage of the immune response suddenly turn into an apoptosis candidate? This is a question that is being investigated by Dr. Rüdiger Arnold. Together with his research team he is studying how the contact of the T cell receptor with the antigen first leads to T cell activation and then switches to AICD shortly afterwards. To elucidate the complex interplay of hundreds of proteins which transmit, modulate, reinforce or block the signals of the T cell receptor within the cell, Arnold and his team are meticulously fitting together one puzzle piece of knowledge after the other.

A key role in this molecular network is played by the NFκB transcription factor, which is normally present in an inactive form in the cytoplasm. After activation by the IκB-Kinase (IKK) enzyme complex , NFκB immediately sets about its work in the nucleus by activating a number of genes that mobilize the immune cells for a defense reaction.

Rüdiger Arnold is focusing on a protein, HPK1 (hematopoietic progenitor kinase 1), which scientists have suspected for some time to influence NFκB activity. The immunologist was able to show that HPK1 acts as a full-length molecule to activate the complex of IκB

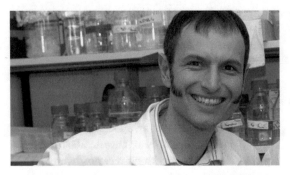

tions through to malignant transformation and cancer. Therefore, it is quite obvious for Arnold which puzzle piece he must fit next into his picture. He is convinced that the question of how an immune response ends cannot be answered without knowing what is regulated by the cleavage of HPK-1.

A Close Look at TCM

kinase, which, in turn, transforms NFκB into its active form. However, shortly after stimulation of the T cell receptor by its antigen, HPK1 is cleaved into two pieces. The resulting molecular fragment, HPK1-C, has exactly opposite functions: It blocks the enzymatic activity of IKK so that NFκB remains in its inactive form. Thus, HPK1-C prevents the reading of genes which maintain the activated state of the T cell and, thus, protect it from apoptosis.

"In principle, a T cell is doomed to die once it has been activated by its antigen, since the T cell receptor/antigen binding promotes the expression of the death ligand, CD95L", Arnold says. "Nevertheless, owing to HPK1, the cells survive at least until they have done their job. Once this protection ends, AICD takes its course."

What would be the consequence if HPK-1 was not cleaved? Surviving T cells could do a great deal of harm in the body – starting from autoimmune reac-

First it was just a hobby that Dr. Min Li-Weber pursued alongside her research on the working mechanisms of messenger substances of the immune system. The Chinese scientist, who came to Germany to do her PhD after graduating in Beijing, is interested in how plant remedies work that are used in the medicine of her home country. For Westerners, the term "traditional Chinese medicine" evokes images of bizarre mixtures of blossoms, leaves and barks, enriched with dried sea-horse, powdered scorpion and mummified tiger penis. It is precisely this concoction image that Min Li-Weber seeks to avoid. She concentrates exclusively on plant constituents that are available as pure substances – as synthetic molecules or isolated from plant extracts. "Traditional Chinese medicine has been used for thousands of years. Over time, doctors were able to gather an enormous body of experience. There is something that makes these traditional remedies particularly interesting to us: They are believed to be mild and low in side effects", the scientist explains. Compounds are often low in side effects if they intervene very selectively and precisely in the biochemical mechanisms of the cell. Li-Weber hopes that such substances, by their mode of action, might point to novel therapeutic targets in the cell. Active ingredients that influence, for example, the complicated signaling cascades of apoptosis or immune regulation, might restore the sensitivity of therapy-resistant tumor cells to cell death.

For her studies, Li-Weber chose plants which Chinese doctors prescribe against tumors and inflammations or which are believed to be generally health-promoting. Among her first candidates there was a medicinal plant that is used as a drug across South-East Asia. Li-Weber chose this plant because earlier investigations had shown that the main constituent of this herb in-

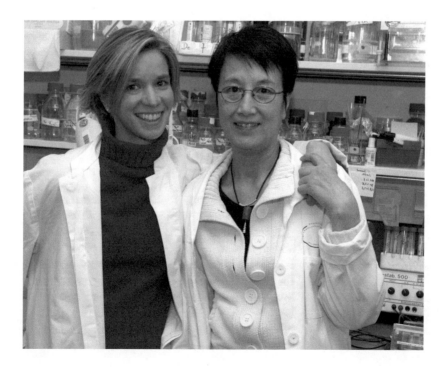

Cell death in the central nervous system or traditional Chinese medicine – what matters is good collaboration

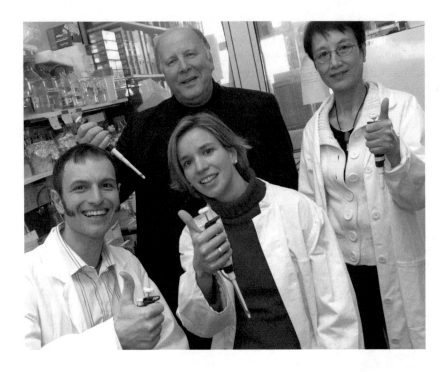

Rüdiger Arnold, Ana Martin-Villalba and Min Li-Weber are part of Peter Krammer's team of approximately 50 staff

duces cell death in bladder and liver cancer cells as well as cells of some leukemias. However, normal white blood cells are left unharmed by the substance.

What causes this selectivity? Li-Weber studied the plant compound in normal and malignant T cells. In the culture dish, the compound induced cell death only in malignant cells, while T cells from healthy donors were not affected – no matter whether they were activated or not.

The substance causes apoptosis in the cancer cells by what is called the intrinsic pathway, in which death receptors such as CD95 do not play a role. Instead, stimuli from within the cell – e.g. in response to stress factors such as radiation or chemotherapy – lead to the release of cytochrome c from the mytochondrial membrane, which triggers the death cascade of the caspases. Another known cause of the intrinsic cell death mechanism is a defective calcium metabolism of the cell. As shown by Li-Weber, this is exactly how the Chinese substance acts in malignant cells. Influenced by the plant component, calcium is released from its intracellular stores into the cytoplasm. It activates a pro-apoptotic protein called Bad, which subsequently induces cell death.

Why does this not happen in healthy cells? "We are working on this", Li-Weber explains. "It may have something to do with the fact that tumor cells have more calcium channels." The result is eagerly awaited, since it this little difference that holds the key for the selectivity and, thus, for the gentle mode of action of the Chinese remedy.

The "Atlas of Chinese Medicinal Plants" is always within reach on the scientist's desk. It is a tome of several hundred pages – there is no lack of candidates from botany. Min Li-Weber is convinced that the herbs from the Middle Kingdom will yet present us with quite a few scientific surprises.

Sibylle Kohlstädt

Literature

Zuliani, C. et al.: Cell Death Differ 13:31, 2006
Brenner, D. et al.: EMBO J 24:4279, 2005
Proksch, P. et al.: J Immunol 174:7075, 2005

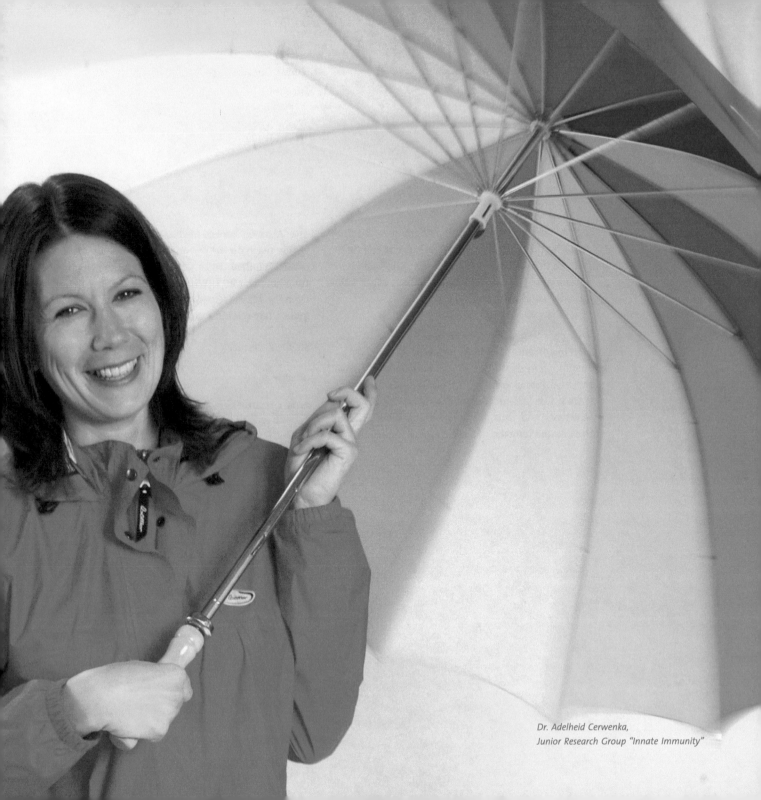

Dr. Adelheid Cerwenka,
Junior Research Group "Innate Immunity"

Born To Be Defense Players: Natural Killer Cells

NK cells are first-line fighters against hostile invaders. They might also be able to defend the organism against tumor cells

The immune system, as our body's own weapon, fights cancer cells. What started out as a highly controversial, even provocative hypothesis in the 1960s, has long since been proven as a fact. The fighters of our immune system attack not only viruses and bacteria. They also recognize and eliminate pathologically transformed cells, often long before these can cause damage by turning into a tumor.

Two closely interacting systems of our body's own defenses are involved in the natural immune response against cancer (see box on p. 104): First, there is the innate immune response, by which invading pathogens or transformed cells are quickly recognized as "foreign" and mostly destroyed. Subsequently, cells of the acquired immune system are activated for fighting off cancer. In contrast to the innate immune system, these go about their job very specifically, targeting specific structures recognized as hostile. The acquired immune system is also responsible for what is called the immunologic memory: In case of a renewed attack by the same attacker, the troops of the acquired

defense system are mounted much more rapidly than at the time of first contact.

To know exactly how defense against tumor cells works is of great importance for cancer research. Once scientists know the mechanisms by which the immune system deals with transformed cells, they will be able to specifically look for ways to mount the body's own defense troops for the fight against cancer. Thus, immune therapy, i.e. specific stimulation of the immune system, may one day become another key pillar of cancer treatment – alongside surgery, radiotherapy and chemotherapy.

Natural Killer Cells As a First Line of Defense

Which fighters of the body's own immune defense lend themselves best to be forged into effective weapons against transformed tissues? "For me and my team, the working mechanisms of natural killer cells are of special interest", says Dr. Adelheid Cerwenka, head of the Theodor Boveri research group "Innate Immunity". Cerwenka, a young scientist, explains in a few words why she attaches so much importance to these blood cells: "One thing is that they are part of the innate immune system and, thus, are able to destroy tumor cells rapidly and directly. In addition, they are capable of activating cells of the acquired immune response so that these also get involved in fighting off cancer."

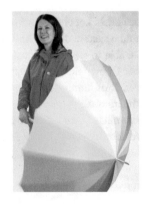

Well shielded from dangers: The immune system protects our body against pathogens – maybe also against cancer?

There is ample evidence suggesting that natural killer (NK) cells attack and eliminate not only infected cells but also tumor cells. For example, scientists have observed in cell culture studies that NK cells are able to kill transformed cells very efficiently. Whether and how well this defense mechanism works in cancer patients is a question that is not easily answered. An afflicted person's immune system is often not strong enough to muster an effective defense against cancer. In addition, in a living organism there is a host of processes going on which can both stimulate and inhibit each other. Therefore, a functioning defense requires not only that the NK cells be at the right place at the right time and recognize tumor tissue. Equally important is that there are no counteracting mechanisms at work that obstruct the killers' work.

Despite all obstacles faced by the immune system in an emergency case, the innate defense against cancer seems to work. Scientists have found first evidence to suggest just this in patients with acute myeloid leukemia following treatment by bone marrow transplant. A donor's bone marrow ensures that the whole range of different blood cells is available in the recipient's organism. The researchers found out that in some patients it is precisely the NK cells which develop an extremely high potential for attacking and eliminating remaining leukemia cells.

Docking Sites for NK Cells

This shows that it is indeed worth taking a closer look at how NK cells fight tumors. In doing so, Cerwenka and her team are trying to answer three big questions: Which signaling pathways cause the cellular killers to become active and join in the combat against cancer? How do NK cells recognize transformed tissue and how can this recognition be improved? How can obstructing processes be suppressed, such as the release of inhibiting substances by cancer cells?

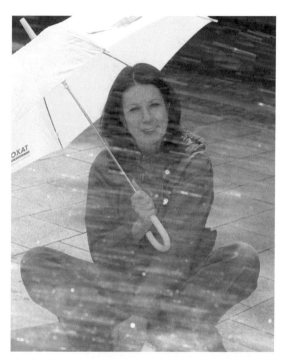

As to tumor recognition, immunologist Cerwenka has laid quite some groundwork jointly with her former co-workers at the DNAX Research Institute in Palo Alto, California. She identified a family of molecules called RAE-1 that are found on the surface of many transformed cells, but not on healthy cells. These structures turned out to be binding partners for a receptor called NKG2D, which NK cells carry on the outside of their cell membrane. Once the NK cells of the immune system have docked at the tumor cells via these recognition structures, they become active and destroy their opponent.

Experiments with mice with transplanted melanoma or lymphoma cells have shown that the efficiency of killer cells increases with the number of RAE-1 recognition molecules they find on the tumor cells. "Therefore, we are searching for signaling pathways that cause cancer cells to form such structures on their surface", explains Cerwenka, adding: "Thus, we might one day be able to make tumors a better target for NK cells."

The Immune System – Defense on Two Fronts

Our body's own defense consists of two different, mutually cooperating systems: the innate immunity and the acquired (also called "adaptive") immunity. The key players in both systems are a multitude of different white blood cells derived from common precursors in the bone marrow. They all pursue one common goal: To defend the organism against invading foreign material and pathogens, but also against transformed body cells.

The cells of the innate immune response act as a first-line defense, often close to the body's entry gates. They are capable of eliminating invaders in a direct manner. Natural killer cells do this by using cell-toxic substances. Other fighters of innate immunity such as macrophages and dendritic cells literally 'eat' the invaders and then display specific characteristic protein segments of the enemy, called antigens, on their cell surface. Embedded in structures called MHC molecules, the antigens are presented to the players of the acquired immune system. Macrophages and dendritic cells are therefore grouped together as antigen-presenting cells.

If the first-line defense alone is not enough to handle an attack, then the acquired immunity gets involved. It is attracted by messenger substances sent out by the cells of the innate immune system and activated by the presented MHC-antigen complexes. Stars of the second-line defense are the B and T lymphocytes. Their common feature is that they are directed exclusively against their "own" antigen in a highly specific way.

After being activated by their antigen, B cells produce antibodies called immunoglobulins. These attach themselves with their specific binding sites to antigen structures of a pathogen, in order to either destroy it directly or prepare it for engulfment by phagocytes – a process called phagocytosis.

Unlike B cells, T cells need the support of antigen-presenting cells. So-called T helper cells support and activate other players of the immune system using various messenger substances. The other group of T lymphocytes kills transformed or virus-infected cells, which is why they are called cytotoxic T cells.

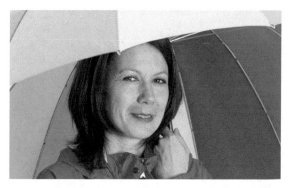

Keeping an Eye on the Opponent

But even if this plan succeeds, it is only a first step. Tumor cells are not without protection against the immune system. In fact, they have developed strategies to evade the defense fighters. "Colleagues in Seattle and Tübingen have found out that soluble binding partners for the NDG2D receptor are found in the blood of patients with various cancers including acute myeloid leukemia. These proteins block the receptor and can thus put killer cells out of action", as DKFZ researcher Cerwenka describes the problem. In addition, cancer cells also release messenger substances such as TGF-β or IL-10, which rob NK cells of their activity.

Therefore, it is not sufficient to look for ways to make tumor tissue more sensitive to attacks by the immune system. We also need to develop strategies to prevent cancer cells from answering the attack by putting killer cells out of action. "Using genetically altered mice, we are planning to take a closer look at both sides of the interaction between tumor cells and NK cells and scrutinize the signaling pathways for potential target sites", summarizes Cerwenka the research project a head of her. She continues: "Thus, we hope that we will soon reach a point where we can intervene and shift the balance towards cancer defense."

Stefanie Reinberger

Literature

Cerwenka, A. et al.: Immunity 12:721, 2000
Cerwenka, A. et al.: PNAS (USA) 98:11521, 2001
Cerwenka, A., Lanier, L.L.: Nature Immunol. Rev 1:41, 2001

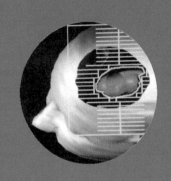

Research Program
Innovative Diagnostics and Therapy

The Research Program is divided into two areas, "Radiological Oncology" and "Experimental Oncology".

Radiological Oncology comprises three research tandems consisting each of one division concerned with fundamental research and one clinically-oriented division or Clinical Cooperation Unit.

The tandem in the area of diagnostic imaging translates experimental studies in the area of high-field magnetic resonance imaging as well as molecular and high resolution imaging into clinical applications.

The tandem in the area of nuclear medicine and molecular imaging evaluates new radiochemical substances for cancer diagnostics.

The tandem in radiation oncology develops and optimizes radiation therapy methods and is internationally acclaimed in the areas of stereotactic radiation therapy, computer-assisted three-dimensional radiotherapy planning, intensity-modulated radiation therapy with inverse radiotherapy planning as well as radiation therapy with carbon ions (heavy ions).

The goal of the divisions in the "Experimental Oncology area is to develop innovative treatment methods on the basis of cells, nucleic acids or antibodies, as well as targeted chemotherapies.

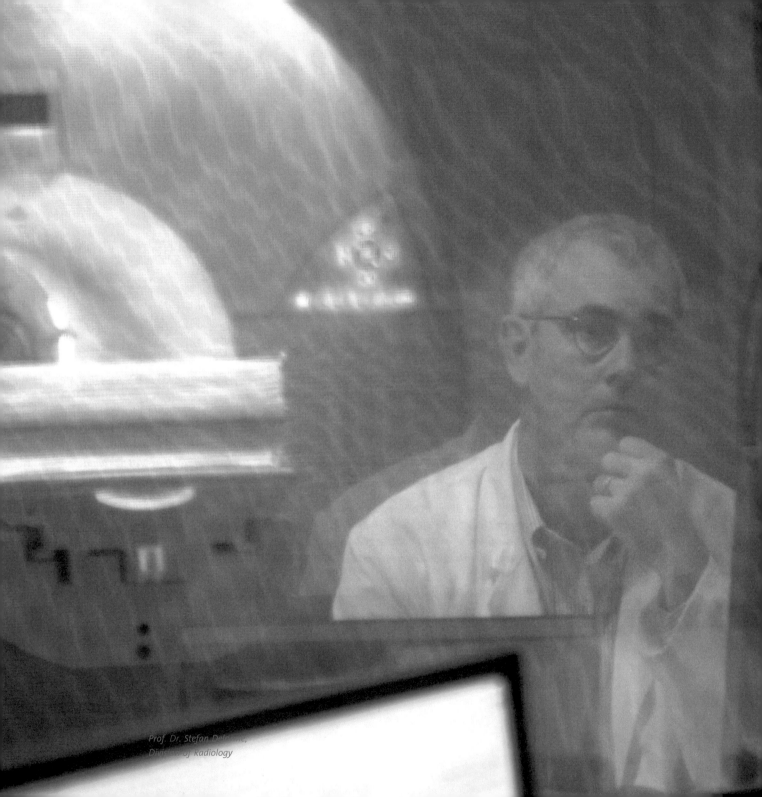

Three Times Magnetic Resonance: Synergic Diagnostics

Will a combination of functional magnetic resonance imaging, dynamic MRI and MR spectroscopy facilitate improved diagnosis of prostate cancer?

It might just be a false alarm. But what if there really is cause for concern? Right now the tumor might still be curable. But what if too much time elapses without action? Perhaps tumor cells will break away and spread within the body. Then again, it might well be benign – and all the fuss about nothing…

An abnormal value in the PSA test, a test used for the early diagnosis of prostate cancer, torments many men with this kind of uncertainty. The test works by determining the concentration in the blood of the prostate-specific antigen, a so-called tumor-marker (see box on p. 111). A value of more than four nanograms per milliliter of blood is considered to be high, but it is not yet proof that a carcinoma is present. If the value is above ten, the doctor will prescribe a biopsy, i.e. the removal of a tissue sample. For results between four and ten a repeat of the PSA test after a few weeks is recommended. If the values are still abnormal, a biopsy is the only course of action.

Other diagnostic procedures are of only limited help to doctors. In ultrasound scans about a third of all prostate cancers remain invisible. Under tactile examination, smaller tumors can only be detected when they are located on the surface of the gland. Even the examination of tissue from the prostate doesn't always provide a clear result: Although samples may be taken systematically from six or eight different points, small tumors can still escape the biopsy needle.

Doctors are reliant upon an unambiguous biopsy result: Both surgical removal of the tumor and therapy with radiation or hormone deprivation are serious interventions; they are not carried out merely on the basis of a suspicion. The PSA value alone is only a hint or an alarm signal, since benign swelling of the prostate or inflammatory processes also often lead to moderately high values of the tumor marker. However, experience shows that, for PSA values in the 'gray area' between four and ten, around a third of the men with negative biopsies are in fact suffering from cancer, not infrequently at a stage that can still be successfully treated. Prostate cancer is only curable provided no cancer cells have become established in the lymph nodes and as long as no distant metastases have developed. The probability that the tumor has already spread increases with increasing PSA value. Thus, when the concentration of tumor marker in the blood lies in the gray region, it is not advisable to wait and keep repeating the test until it unambiguously indicates the presence of a tumor.

Prostate cancer, with about 32,000 new cases diagnosed each year in Germany is the most common malignant disease among men. This number makes clear the scale of the problem.

In 2002, Professor Stefan Delorme of the Radiology Division and his coworker Dr. Christian Zechmann began a prospective study in collaboration with the Urological University Hospital in Mannheim. The doctors wanted to establish whether, in cases of suspected prostate cancer, a combination of different magnetic resonance imaging techniques is able to yield a reliable diagnosis faster and more directly. The study participants were men with a doubtful PSA value, i.e. in the range 4 to 15, but whose biopsy result was negative.

One Machine, Three Methods of Analysis

"A single diagnostic procedure that can detect prostate cancer with one-hundred percent certainty does not exist and will not become available for the fore seeable future", says Delorme. "So we are tackling the diagnosis problem – little by little – via a different approach. We combine three different methods. Each on its own is frequently incapable of telling us with certainty whether a malignant transformation has occurred. But we are putting our money on the synergy effects of the combination."

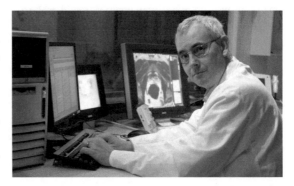

PSA Test: Pros and Cons

The PSA test, introduced at the end of the 1980s as a method of early diagnosis of prostate cancer, determines the concentration of the prostate-specific antigen in the blood. This is an enzyme which helps to liquefy the semen, thus contributing to the mobility of the sperm. Although healthy prostate tissue also produces PSA, the protein is suited as a tumor marker since cancer cells produce a significantly larger amount. Whilst PSA screening is widely used in the USA, in Germany it is not one of the methods covered by the health insurance within the framework of early cancer diagnosis. Here it is only carried out if a man explicitly requests it. This rule is controversial. On the one hand, it has been demonstrated that PSA tests enable more cancers to be recognized at an early stage than is possible with tactile examination alone. However, it is not yet clear whether this leads to a decrease in mortality. It is currently the topic of large prospective studies such as the European Randomized Study of Screening for Prostate Cancer (ERSPC). In 2005, a smaller case control study with a lower epidemiological predictive value was published. It indicated that the mortality rate due to advanced prostate cancer could be reduced by 35% with the test.

Critics of a PSA screening object that the test leads to the discovery of numerous small and only slightly malignant tumors that really don't call for treatment. If in such cases the man decides to undergo an operation or radiation therapy, the damage could well be greater than the benefit.

The guidelines of the German urologists thus recommend that patients are informed in detail about the possible consequences before a PSA test is carried out.

The basis for all three techniques that Delorme uses is magnetic resonance. Magnetic resonance imaging (MRI) is familiar as a sort of radiation-free x-ray. The Heidelberg radiologists, however, are using the technique not only to generate images of the inside of the body: they also combine it with two further methods of analysis, dynamic MRI and magnetic resonance spectroscopy.

Magnetic resonance spectroscopy utilizes the fact that protons, the nuclei of hydrogen atoms, behave like tiny magnets. Under normal circumstances they are completely randomly oriented in tissue. However, in a strong magnetic field, a small fraction of them reorients in the direction of the applied field, in much the same way as a compass needle orients itself in the Earth's magnetic field. These protons are able to temporarily absorb and then re-radiate the energy of radio waves of a precisely defined frequency. An antenna, known as a solenoid, present in the housing of the equipment or brought into close contact with the prostate via a probe inserted into the rectum, emits the radio waves and simultaneously receives the signal produced by the protons. How rapidly and with what intensity the protons emit their signal depends on what molecules are present in their immediate vicinity. A contrast agent containing the element gadolinium has a particularly strong influence on the signal. Injected into the blood, it becomes distributed throughout the body and amplifies the proton signal.

Depending on the information required, there are different ways of evaluating the MR signals. Delorme uses the so-called T2-weighted measurement to generate the familiar images of the tissue. In these images carcinomas appear darker than the surrounding tissue. "But this is only valid for the so-called peripheral zone of the prostate", says Delorme, qualifying the former statement. Here, however, is where most carcinomas arise; most growths found in the inner region of the organ are benign. What is dangerous are the rare cases in which a tumor develops in the inner region, where it is invisible in the T2-weighted imaging.

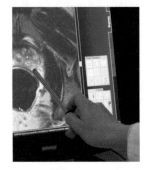

The contrast agent gadolinium enhances the imaging of tissues

Blood Flow in Tumor Made Visible

A different kind of information is obtained from dynamic magnetic resonance imaging. This technique gives information about the flow of blood in the tissue under study. In order to grow, tumors have to attract blood vessels, which grow into the tumor and supply its needs. The density of blood vessels in tumor tissue is usually higher than in healthy tissue. The walls of these arteries are often 'leaky' so that blood can seep out of the vessels and into the intercellular spaces in the tumor. These differences in the vascularization and the vessel wall permeability are imaged by dynamic MRI. For the analysis, the doctors use a complicated mathematical procedure, which represents the rate of exchange of blood between the vascular system and the 'interstitial' space, i.e. the spaces between the cells. The rate of exchange is a measure

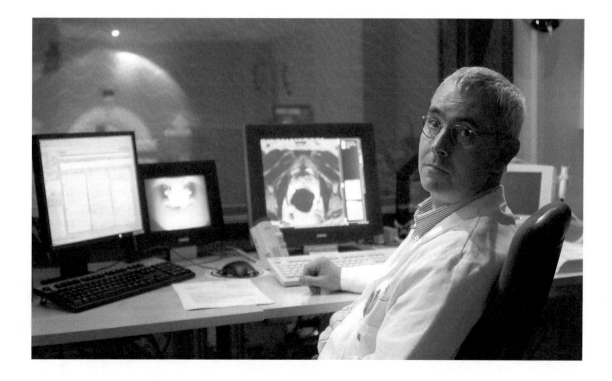

of the velocity with which the fluid from the larger vessels penetrates the tissue. Less complicated, but just as precise in the results it yields, is a plot of the curve representing the signal increase with time. The radiologists have observed that the rise of the amplified MR signal with contrast agent is different for normal tissue and for tumor tissue. Whilst in healthy tissue the signal rises slowly after about one minute and then remains for quite a while at its maximum level, in tumor tissue it rises rapidly but then falls again significantly after about two minutes. This behavior of the signals is already known from breast cancer.

Further diagnostic certainty is achieved with MR spectroscopy, which images the metabolic properties of the tissue. The procedure detects characteristic biomolecules. In their study, the doctors are concentrating on choline and citrate. Choline is an important constituent of the lipid molecules in the cell membrane. In tumor cells, which, because of their high rate of division, continually demand new membrane, the level of choline is raised. Citrate is one of the numerous molecules secreted by the prostate into the seminal fluid. In tumors, which have often lost the physiological properties of their original tissue, the levels of citrate generally sink. A comparison of the concentration of these two indicator molecules often reveals regions of suspect tissue in the gland.

Targeted Biopsies, Gentler Therapies

"Our primary aim", says Stefan Delorme, "is to provide urologists with a kind of navigational aid for carrying out biopsies. If our data indicate a suspect region, they can – with the help of ultrasound – target this area and take a tissue sample which yields a reliable diagnosis."

So far, the Mannheim hospital and urologists in private practice have sent about 150 patients to the DKFZ for MRI. Delorme and Zechmann estimate that in about a year they will have assembled enough data to perform a statistical evaluation of their study. This will tell us just how accurately the elaborate triple diagnostics can guide the biopsy needle to the tumor.

Stefan Delorme hopes that the combined MR examinations will not only contribute to more reliable diagnoses, but simultaneously pave the way towards a more targeted radiation therapy of prostate cancers. The radiologist expects that triple MR diagnostics may be able to differentiate between tumor regions of different aggressiveness. With modern radiation techniques such as IMRT (see box on p. 119), it is possible to deliver a high radiation dose to a tumor area that is growing with particular malignance. It is still the case that the entire prostate will have to be irradiated, since small tumor nodules that are too small to be detected with MRI are frequently distributed throughout the organ. But very close to the prostate lies the radiation-sensitive rectum, and here too are the nerve bundles that regulate the erection capability. If one can concentrate a high radiation dose onto the most aggressive region of the tumor, it will be possible, while achieving a higher rate of cure, to better protect these sensitive tissues.

Sibylle Kohlstädt

Literature

Kiessling, F. et al.: Radiologe 43:474, 2003
Kiessling, F. et al.: Eur. Radiol. 14:1793, 2004

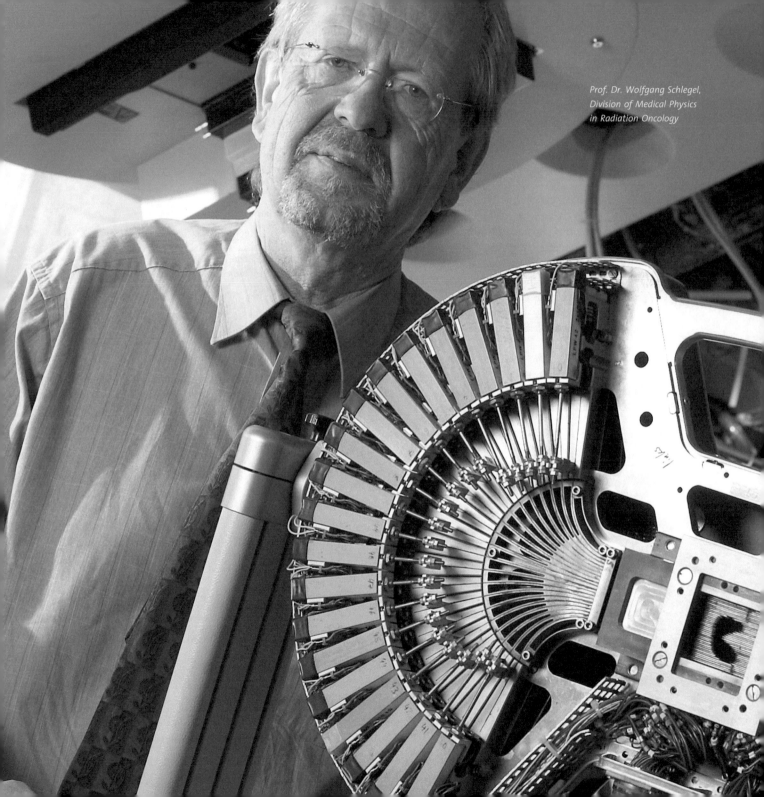

Prof. Dr. Wolfgang Schlegel,
Division of Medical Physics
in Radiation Oncology

Radiation with Insight

On many weekends there is a surprising amount of activity in the basement of the DKFZ: Behind meter-thick concrete walls a group of physicists, engineers and doctors are busy taking apart a makeshift-looking machine, the experimental linear accelerator. The individual parts of the machine are needed on the ground floor for the radiation equipment used to treat patients. There the scientists are mounting an x-ray tube and installing a radiation detector. Thick bundles of cables have to be laid and all the components of the apparatus must be re-adjusted. The job has to be completed without delay so as not to interfere with the packed plan of patient appointments. It goes without saying that the staff of the Division of Medical Physics in Radiation Oncology are prepared to give up their Saturdays and Sundays for this. After nearly four days' installation, an officer from the German safety standards authority TÜV finally has to approve the reconstruction.

The reason for this time-consuming effort is to facilitate tests of a new method of treatment. The scientists are preparing the radiation equipment – the linear accelerator, linac for short – for use in 'image-guided' or 'adaptive' radiotherapy.

In their work, radiotherapists are confronted with a continually recurring problem: Their success in curing cancer improves when they increase the dose of radiation administered to the tumor. But, the higher the dose, the more essential it becomes to avoid irradiation of the surrounding healthy tissue. Thanks to new procedures, radiotherapy has achieved an unbelievable degree of precision in recent years (see box on p. 119). Today, therapists can direct the beam onto the tumor with an accuracy of half a millimeter. But what if the tumor isn't actually located at the position assumed by the doctors, or if its position changes during the treatment?

...Control Is Better

With the new method developed by the Deutsches Krebsforschungszentrum, which combines linear accelerator and x-ray computer tomography in a single machine, it is possible to check the tumor location whenever necessary.

"Our technique is ideal in that it allows doctors to quickly obtain a picture of the actual situation before the start of each therapy cycle", says Professor Wolfgang Schlegel, head of the Division of Medical Physics in Radiation Oncology. Schlegel's motivation for developing this new method came from a longstanding problem in radiotherapy: Many tumors shift their position as a result of involuntary movements in the body. A good example is prostate cancer: Depending on how full the bladder is the position of the tumor can vary by as much as one centimeter. But particularly for the prostate the greatest care is needed, since it lies immediately next to the rectum, which is extremely sensitive to radiation and should always receive as little as possible. For other cancers it is the therapy itself that causes changes in the volume and the shape of the tumor, for example in cases where the radiation successfully causes tumors in the head and neck region to shrink. From the time of the imaging diagnosis, which is used to plan the radiation therapy, to the completion of up to 38 therapy cycles, several weeks if not months will elapse. Clearly it is better if the doctors do not have to rely only on their original images.

Other members of Schlegel's division are also involved in the development of the adaptive therapy, namely the physicists Dr. Bernd Hesse, Professor Uwe Oelfke, Dr. Simeon Nill and Thomas Tücking, as well as the engineer Gernot Echner. For producing the images the scientists employ a strongly divergent conical x-ray beam. This yields an image of the entire radiation region, using a single sweep of the x-ray tube around

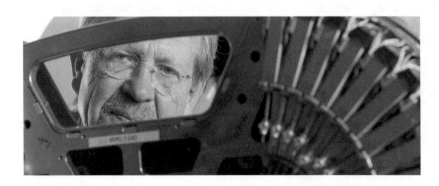

The multileaf collimator, which acts as a radiation screen, adapts the therapy beam to the individual tumor anatomy

Sensitive Organs Increasingly Spared

Many technical innovations have contributed in recent decades to make radiotherapy more effective and simultaneously gentler. Today, over 60 percent of all cancer patients undergo radiotherapy with the aim of achieving a complete cure or a significant relief of suffering. About 50 percent of all cancer patients can now be cured. In about one half of these cases, radiotherapy contributes to the successful treatment, either as the sole therapy or in combination with surgery and/or chemotherapy.

Professor Wolfgang Schlegel and the staff of his division at the German Cancer Research Center have made a major contribution to this progress. They are responsible, among other things, for the development of the multileaf collimator, a screen that is positioned in front of the accelerator and whose computer controlled lamellae, or leaves, are used to shape the cross-section of the beam. In this way the beam, regardless of its incident angle, can be adapted to the contour of the tumor; this method is known as conformal radiation therapy. But for tumors with a complicated shape, even this method has its limits. In the ideal case the dose administered to the tumor is so high that all cancer cells are destroyed. But this is difficult to achieve when malignant tumors have grown around sensitive organs, such as the optic nerve or the spinal cord, in the shape of a horseshoe, meaning that sensitive tissue is necessarily in the firing line of the radiation. Here one can exploit another invention of Schlegel's division, intensity modulated radiation therapy (IMRT). This method is based on the modulation of the radiation dose within a radiation field. In this way it is possible to increase the dose within the tumor without causing collateral damage to sensitive neighboring organs. IMRT requires a completely new kind of therapy planning. The optimum dose distribution is no longer established by the doctor by trying out various intensities and incident angles. Instead he gives the computer the information about the tumor contours and about sensitive neighboring organs, about the desired dose in the tumor and the tolerance dose in the sensitive organs. The computer then calculates the optimum dose distribution (reverse planning).

Various studies are already demonstrating advantages for the patient: In the case of prostate cancer, the incidence of intestinal complications decreases; for breast cancer, the heart and lungs are spared, and for the treatment of head and neck tumors, the salivary glands benefit. IMRT is now in employed in many hospitals throughout the world.

the patient's body. A detector plate made of amorphous silicon, positioned opposite the x-ray tube, records one or two images for every degree of rotation. The process takes about one minute. In almost no time at all the computer reconstructs from these individual images a three-dimensional view of the tumor which is displayed on the monitor.

A special feature of this prototype equipment from the German Cancer Research Center is the 180° arrangement of the components: the accelerator and the x-ray tube are directly opposite one another. This ensures that even tiny lateral displacements of the tumor out of the radiation field are recorded. Small displacements in the perpendicular direction, however, are of no great significance for the accuracy and safety of the treatment.

Since the end of 2004, image-guided radiotherapy is being clinically tested at the DKFZ. The radiotherapists

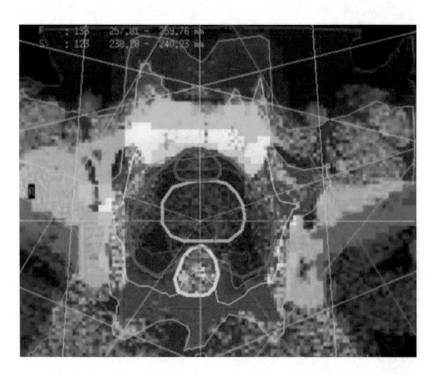

In computer-assisted radiotherapy planning, isodoses are indicated by colored lines

are using the conical beam to ascertain the perfect positioning for a number of patients with a variety of cancers. Each of these treatments requires the prior time-consuming conversion of the accelerator, and every time the machine has to be approved by the TÜV.

Relief for Patients

In future, patients should benefit from not only safer but also better tolerable radiotherapy. In order to make the most of the potential offered by the high accuracy of a precision radiotherapy, it is necessary today to rigidly fix patients to the treatment table. For patients with tumors in the head or neck, who are treated at the German Cancer Research Center with intensity modulated radiotherapy, this involves squeezing into a close-fitting, individually made plastic mask for each therapy session. Only the tip of the nose remains free for breathing. If a prostate carcinoma is being treated, in addition to the head mask, the patient must also wear a body-corset, which is screwed to the treatment table. If, however, it is possible to visually follow the tumor in every radiotherapy session so that the positioning can be correspondingly re-adjusted – 'adapted' – then there is no need to constrain the patients in the way just described. This is a great relief – and not only for persons who suffer from claustrophobia. It represents an increase in the comfort of patients and, in the long term, also reduces costs: the manufacture of individual masks and body corsets is time-consuming and requires specially trained medical personnel.

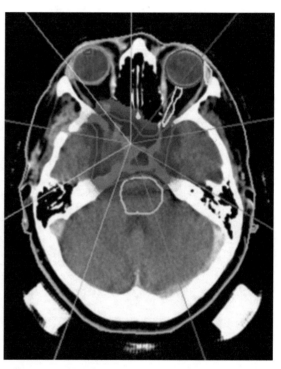

The lines correspond to the incident angles

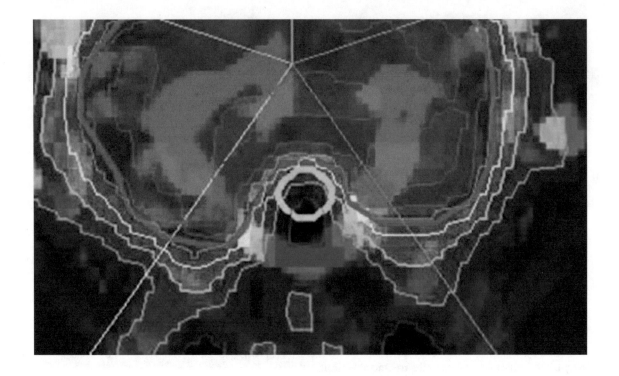

Tumors under Permanent Visual Control

In addition to the control and re-adjustment that it
makes possible, this new technology is considered by
doctors to have further quite different areas of application: They are thinking about a cancer treatment in
which the beam of radiation is only switched on
when the tumor intersects its path. This form of treatment, known as 'gated therapy', is currently being set
up at the DKFZ for the treatment of lung cancer.
A sensor belt around the ribcage monitors the
patient's respiratory frequency and movement. At
the same time one can follow how the lung tumor
shifts with the up and down of the breathing.
The aim is to synchronize the therapy beam with
the movement in such a way that the beam is fired
at the exact moment when the tumor is in
a particular position.

"We hope that this will bring lung-cancer patients greater benefit from radiotherapy", says Professor Peter Huber, head of the Clinical Cooperation Unit Radiation Oncology, "because until now the risk of further damaging the sensitive lung tissue was too high." Patients with tumors of the pancreas or liver metastases, which are likewise displaced with the breathing, could also benefit from this movement-synchronized irradiation.

What is the vision of the radiotherapists? The best thing would be if one never lost sight of the tumor, says Wolfgang Schlegel. He is referring here to continual visual tracking of the tumor through the path of the beam. But for this to be possible, a few technical hurdles still have to be overcome. "The development of image-guided therapy is still in its infancy", notes Schlegel, "both in terms of its technical realization and in relation to its fields of application." The potential of this invention from Schlegel's division has already been recognized elsewhere: The company Siemens Medical Solutions has purchased a licence for this technology from the Deutsches Krebsforschungszentrum and intends to bring the equipment on the market worldwide.

Sybille Kohlstädt

Literature

Oelfke, U. et al.: Medical Dosimetry 31(1), 2006
Nill, S. et al.: Phys Med Biol 50:4087, 2005

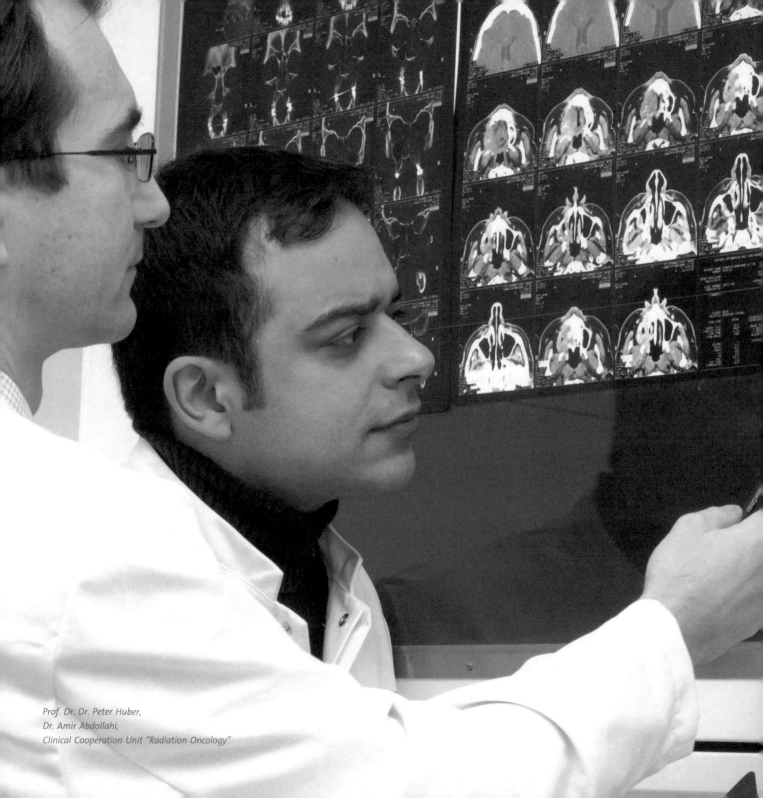

Prof. Dr. Dr. Peter Huber,
Dr. Amir Abdollahi,
Clinical Cooperation Unit "Radiation Oncology"

Trimodal Approach Puts the Screws on the Tumor

The Fourth Pillar?

Substances that inhibit the formation of new vessels enhance the effectiveness of a combination of radiotherapy and chemotherapy

One millimeter in cross-section. No bigger than a pinhead. This is the maximum size almost any tumor can reach if it does not get connected to the supply channels of the blood vessels. Tumors, like any other tissue, need a supply of nutrients and oxygen through blood. They initiate their own supply: Induced by a lack of oxygen or gene mutations, they start producing protein factors that promote the sprouting of blood vessels and attract them to the tumor. The formation of new vessels, or angiogenesis, is vital for tumor growth and, thus, a potential Achilles' heel of a tumor. Oncologists are currently placing great hopes on blocking this process.

Professor Peter Huber leads the Clinical Cooperation Unit "Radiation Oncology" at the German Cancer Research Center. Collaborating with colleagues from "Medical Physics", Huber and his coworkers are developing and testing novel precision radiotherapy treatments (see article on page 117). Using the new techniques of precise and gentle radiotherapy, partly in

combination with chemotherapy, it is today possible to cure substantially more patients than about 20 years ago. The goal of Peter Huber and his colleagues is to further increase the rate of cure. They are searching for new approaches, additional strategies, that might add a fourth option to the traditional three "pillars" of cancer treatment – surgery, radiotherapy, chemotherapy. And they are searching for therapeutic possibilities to make existing treatment approaches more effective and reduce side effects.

Why are radiation therapists targeting angiogenesis? "Radiation causes a vehement reaction of the tumor", says Peter Huber. "In this process, numerous cellular repair mechanisms are started. Among other things, the cancer cells release large amounts of angiogenesis factors to save their vital blood vessels. This is what we try to counteract."

The most important angiogenesis factor is VEGF, which acts on the inner lining of blood vessels, the endothelial cells. Binding of VEGF to its receptor on the endothelial cell membrane marks the start of a cas-

cade of biochemical signals that eventually lead to activation of angiogenesis. A high VEGF level in tumors
correlates with a high density of blood vessels. This,
in turn, is associated with a poor prognosis and resistance to radiation therapy, at least for some types of
cancer.

Triple Approach Is More Effective

Professor Huber, his colleague Dr. Amir Abdollahi and
coworkers recently demonstrated for the first time
that blocking of angiogenesis can improve the effectiveness of a standard therapy approach. In experiments with cell cultures and mice, they compared a
combination of radiotherapy and the chemotherapy
drug Pemetrexed with a triple approach, in which an
angiogenesis inhibitor, SU11657, was administered in
addition. The substance blocked the tyrokinase activity of the VEGF receptor and, thus, prevented in the

endothelial cells that the signaling cascade leading to
the formation of new vessels was triggered.

No matter which tumor parameters the scientists investigated – the trimodal treatment always showed
better results: Tumor cells grew more slowly, endothelial cells were increasingly forced to commit suicide.
In their experiments with animals, too, the triple
approach proved to be superior: In mice with transplanted human skin tumors, the cancer cells under triple attack were less able to grow invasively into
neighboring muscle tissue than in conventionally
treated animals.

The trimodal approach works best if the angiogenesis
inhibitor is administered prior to the other two treatments. This is probably so, because SU11657 can thus
counteract the angiogenesis-promoting effect of radiotherapy – the release of VEGF – from the very beginning. But the scientists demonstrated two more rea-

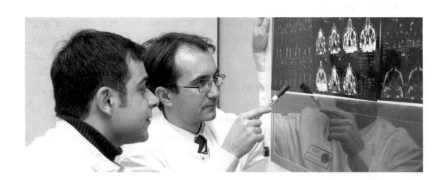

Radiotherapy planning is always based on imaging technologies such as computed tomography or magnetic resonance imaging

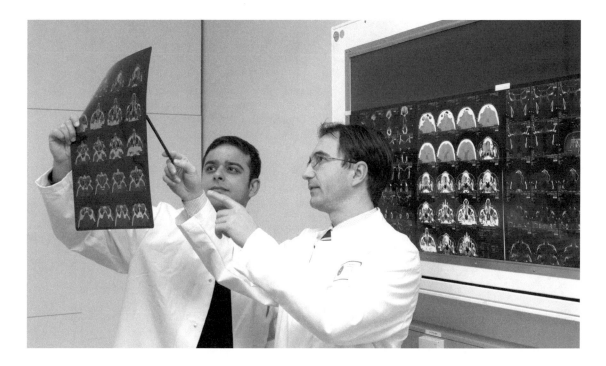

sons for the success of their trimodal treatment approach: Chemotherapy and radiation therapy cause programmed cell death in tumor cells. One of the survival strategies of tumors is to escape this death signal by activating a protection molecule called Akt. This biochemical escape also seems to be prevented by SU11657. In addition, a tumor reacts to irradiation by making vessel walls permeable. Fluid then passes from the blood vessels into the tissue where it leads to an elevated interstitial pressure. The pressure in-crease leads to a reduced blood flow in the tumor tissue. The consequences: Cytotoxins no longer get to their destination, and there is a lack of oxygen. This, in turn, reduces the effectiveness of radiotherapy, which is based not only on direct damage to DNA, but also on the formation of toxic oxygen radicals. SU11657 reduces the pressure within the tumor by more than one half in one day, possibly because it counteracts the permeability of the blood vessels. The substance seems to attack the tumor from all sides.

Resistant to Resistances

What makes angiogenesis such an attractive target for novel treatment approaches? Anti-angiogenesis as a treatment does not target the genetically instable tumor cells, but the endothelial cells of the blood vessels. Attracted by growth factors of the tumor, they are the origin of new blood capillaries.

Many sophisticated strategies of attacking tumors fail because of the extremely high mutation rate of cancer cells: If a drug interferes with a tumor-specific metabolic pathway, a mutation of a single enzyme is often enough to make the drug attack ineffective. Other tissues with high cell division rates do not respond so rapidly by resistance formation. Thus, bone marrow cells and hair follicles die with each new chemotherapy cycle even if the tumor against which the treatment is directed has long since ceased to respond to the cytotoxins. Therefore, doctors hope that the new strategy will help achieve sustained, or at least prolonged, effectiveness.

A first hint to this effect was provided in 1997 by US scientists. In experiments with mice, they were able to show that endostatin, an endogenous inhibitor of angiogenesis, did not lose its effectiveness in various tumors even after six subsequent cycles of treatment. The bright promise of therapeutic use of endostatin, which is formed during proteolytic cleavage of the cytoskeleton protein (collagen), has not been fulfilled

yet. However, a whole range of synthetic or gene-technologically produced angiogenesis inhibitors have become available since then. Most of these substances target the key reaction of the process, i.e. binding of the growth factor VEGF to its receptor on the surface of endothelial cells. These inhibitors can largely be grouped in two categories: antibodies directed against VEGF and low-molecular inhibitors of VEGF receptor tyrosine kinase.

A VEGF antibody with the trade name Avastin received approval for treatment of metastatic colorectal cancer in 2004. A whole range of antiangiogenic substances for use in treating breast and renal cell cancer, glioblastoma, melanoma and others are in late stages of clinical testing. The drug Thalidomide, which became sadly famous under the trade name Contergan, has been used successfully against multiple myeloma. Thalidomide also inhibits the formation of new vessels, but the working mechanisms are not entirely clarified yet.

Despite the joy at the success of the new drugs we must consider that angiogenesis inhibitors do not act cytotoxically but cytostatically. They only put tumors and metastases in a kind of dormant state and, thus, theoretically need to be taken lifelong. Whether the substances remain effective if taken over decades is yet unknown.

Clinical Trials in Preparation

With multi-modal treatment concepts, oncologists hope not only to increase effectiveness, but also to lessen side effects. Additional treatment with angiogenesis inhibitors does not appear to further increase the toxicity of the treatment. Doctors hope that it might even be possible to reduce the cytotoxin doses in weakened patients, who are not able to cope with the severe side effects of some chemotherapy drugs.

After the promising preclinical results of the trimodal treatment concept, there are plans to start clinical testing as soon as possible. Peter Huber plans to conduct a first trial in collaboration with the Department of Radiation Oncology and Radiation Therapy of Heidelberg University Radiological Hospital and the University Surgical Hospital. Heidelberg has evolved into a nationally recognized center for the treatment of pancreatic cancer – a type of cancer that urgently re-

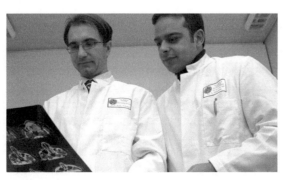

quires enhanced treatment concepts. Therefore, the first 20 patients with advanced stages of pancreatic cancer have already been included in the trial.

Some cancer treatments do not need increased effectiveness. But it would help many patients if it were possible to reduce the adverse effects on health through treatment. Among the most severe and life-threatening side effects of cancer treatment is pulmonary fibrosis, a condition that can develop as a result of radiation therapy or chemotherapy of lung cancer. It involves proliferation of fibrous connective tissue and gradually leads to hardening of the lung tissue so that breathing becomes increasingly restricted. In the worst case, the disease is terminal.

Researchers in Huber's division have elucidated the molecular causes behind the development of this condition. They started out with the assumption that here, too, radiation induces a release of growth factors. Experiments with cells in the culture dish showed that they were right: Following irradiation, high levels of the PDGF growth factor, a close relative of VEGF, were found in the culture medium.

Kinase Inhibitor Stops Fibrosis

Based on this result, the researchers came up with a strategy for therapeutic intervention. Fibroblasts carry the PDGF receptor on their membrane. The receptor binding promotes cell growth and thus induces fibro-

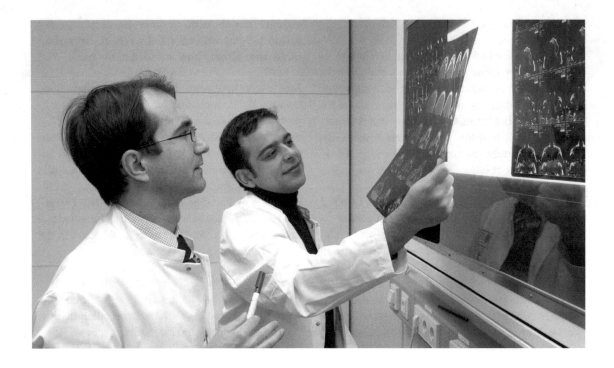

sis formation. Similar to the VEGF receptor, the target molecule of PDGF is a receptor tyrosine kinase. This means that inhibitors of kinase activity should be capable of counteracting the disease process.

This hypothesis has now been proven in mice that had been received high radiation doses. Animals that had been treated with one of three different kinase inhibitors (SU9518, SU11657 and Imatinib/Glivec) survived significantly longer than untreated animals.

Both CT and histological examinations revealed less signs of fibrosis in the lungs of the treated animals.

"This encourages us to test kinase inhibitors in patients receiving radiation therapy", says Peter Huber, commenting the results. In 20 to 30 percent of lung cancer patients fibrotic developments prevent treating tumors with sufficiently high radiation doses. Protection by the new substances might allow one to apply the necessary radiation doses to the tumor and, thus, to improve the chances of cure for patients. The researchers anticipate that the drugs might also be useful for treating spontaneous fibrosis.

The good news is that these findings might be used for the benefit of patients with unusual swiftness. Glivec, one of the three kinase inhibitors studied, has already passed all stages of drug approval and has been used in clinical practice for treating certain types of leukemias and tumors of the gastrointestinal tract. Jointly with the Heidelberg Thorax Clinic and the University Radiological Hospital, Peter Huber plans to study soon whether addition of Glivec to radiotherapy protects against the dangerous side effect of lung cancer radiation treatment.

Sibylle Kohlstädt

Literature

Abdollahi, A. et al.: J Exp Med 201:925, 2005
Huber, P. et al.: Cancer Res. 65:3643, 2005
Abdollahi, A. et al.: Molecular Cell 13:649, 2004

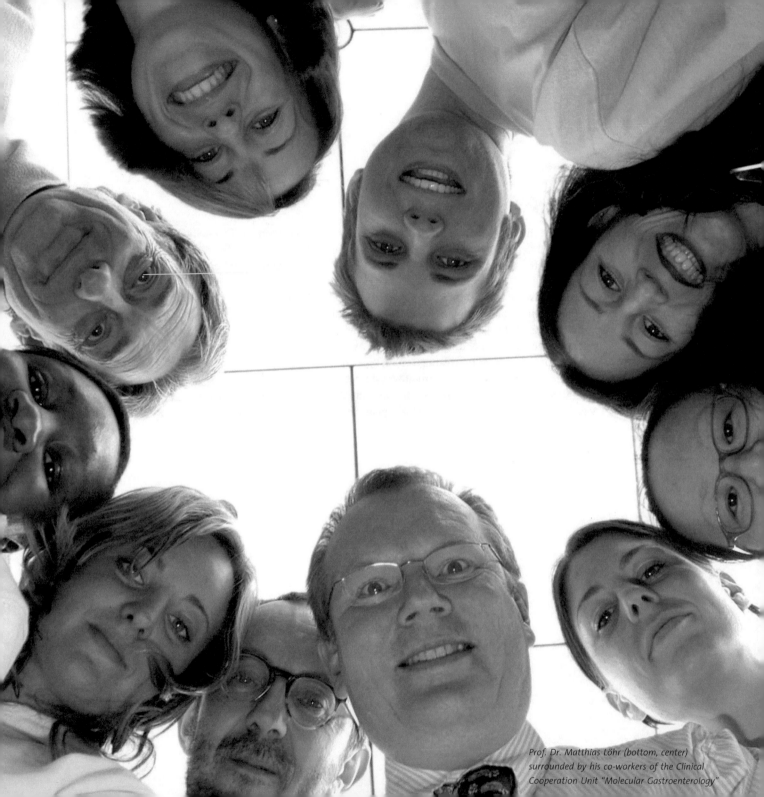

Prof. Dr. Matthias Löhr (bottom, center) surrounded by his co-workers of the Clinical Cooperation Unit "Molecular Gastroenterology"

Smuggled in Special Capsules

A combination of chemotherapy and gene therapy provides good results in the treatment of pancreatic cancer

Although gene therapy has been a long-running hit in the media, success reports have been rare so far. In Mannheim, however, the method is already employed for the benefit of patients: Professor Matthias Löhr, head of the Clinical Cooperation Unit "Molecular Gastroenterology" at the University Hospitals in Mannheim, uses a combination of gene therapy and chemotherapy to treat a rare, but extremely dangerous type of cancer. Cancer of the pancreas, or pancreatic carcinoma in technical terms, is diagnosed each year in one in ten thousand people in Germany. The disease is associated with a very poor prognosis. Barely ten percent of sufferers survive the first year after diagnosis.

The problem is that pancreatic carcinoma is usually not detected before a very late stage. It does not cause any symptoms for a long time, and when it does, symptoms are very unspecific. Thus, the mostly elderly patients complain about loss of appetite or nausea, they lose weight or suffer from pain in the back and in the abdomen. Reduced fitness, diarrhea and itching also belong to the list of unspecific symptoms.

Late Diagnosis – Poor Prognosis

Until the real cause of discomfort is found, the tumor has time to grow. Due to the anatomic location on the posterior abdominal wall it also has ample room to spread undetected for a long time. In addition, tumor cells take advantage of the arteries running directly along or even in the pancreas. Thus, they quickly gain access to the blood supply, which again promotes tumor growth. Moreover, pancreatic carcinomas tend to spread along nerve tracts and in lymphatic vessels. This makes surgery extremely difficult; only one in five tumors can be surgically removed at all. In 90 percent of patients the tumor at the time of diagnosis has already grown to such a size and has invaded other tissues to an extent that makes complete removal impossible.

But not only surgery usually fails as a treatment option. Radiation therapy and chemotherapy are also often ineffective due to the resistance of the tumors. Moreover, with the tumor's location deep inside the body, radiation frequently is more damaging than helpful. "Even though therapeutic radiation can be aimed very precisely today, it is almost unavoidable that healthy tissue gets damaged, too – particularly when the tumor is hidden like that", Löhr explains.

A Comeback of an Old Drug

Back in the mid-sixties, a drug called ifosfamide was developed, with the first ever use in clinical practice in 1971. The substance has shown a certain effectiveness against tumors of the pancreas, although in high dosages only. While children cope relatively well with ifosfamide treatment, the majority of patients with pancreatic cancer are elderly people, who suffer from severe side effects. "But since cancer medicine also follows the principle that therapy should never put more strain on a patient than the disease itself, ifosfamide was abandoned for treating pancreatic cancer back in the early nineties", says Matthias Löhr, describing the consequences.

Yet, searching for an innovative treatment approach, the medical researcher and his team once more came across the drug which had really been written off in terms of pancreatic cancer. "Ifosfamide is of interest for us, because it is a so-called prodrug, i.e. a drug that is administered in an inactive form and is then turned into an effective agent in the body", says Löhr to describe what is special about the anticancer agent. The key role in the activation of the substance is played by an enzyme called cytochrome P450, whose normal

task is to dispose of toxic substances in the body. Transformation of the ifosfamide prodrug in the body also means: The drug can only be as effective as it is metabolized in the body. And since it is metabolized almost exclusively in the liver, its active variant reaches the pancreas from there only systemically, i.e., via the bloodstream. This is why in the early treatment trials the substance needed to be given in such high dosages and caused such severe side effects.

Trying to solve this problem, Löhr had an idea: If it were possible to transform ifosfamide into its active variant directly in the pancreas to be treated, its efficacy should improve – and at lower dosages, too. For without the detour via the liver, one could reach a higher concentration directly at the tumor without putting too much strain on the whole organism.

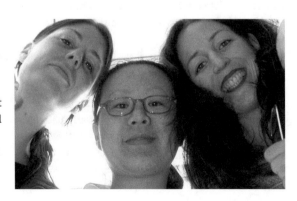

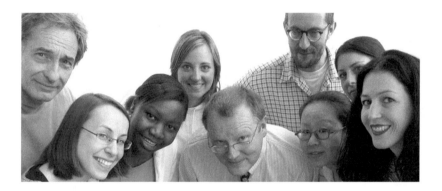

More Than Just Packaging

The solution was a combination of chemotherapy and gene therapy. Löhr and his coworkers selected a human cell line that had already proven useful in many therapy studies. They manipulated the cells in such a way that they produce large amounts of cytochrome CYP2B1. Then the cells thus equipped were enclosed into small cellulose capsules – a technique originally developed by the Institute of Polymer Research in Rostock. Thus encapsulated, the cells are not recognized by the immune system and therefore not attacked. In the pancreas, the small packages support the metabolization of the chemotherapy drug. Ifosfamide enters the capsules through microscopically small pores and is transformed there into its active form by the enclosed cells. The active product enters the pancreatic tissue by the same way and does its therapeutic work.

At the same time, the genetically manipulated cells stay safely stored away inside the polymer capsules.

The first "study subjects" used by the scientist for testing the new treatment approach were nude mice whom he had injected tumor cells under the skin. After the tumor had grown, the animals were injected the capsules directly into the tumor and received a systemic ifosfamide therapy. He achieved the desired result: Thanks to the encapsulated cells, the efficacy of ifosfamide had increased to such an extent that the tumors had shrunk significantly in all the animals after three weeks of treatment. In 20 percent of the mice the tumors had disappeared completely.

Valuable Aid in Pancreatic Surgery

For planning surgery of a pancreatic carcinoma, it is vital that surgeons know the exact anatomic conditions around the tumor. The pancreas is tightly embedded between the intestine, liver, spleen, and stomach; vital large blood vessels are located in the immediate vicinity. Scientists of the Division of Medical and Biological Informatics of the Deutsches Krebsforschungszentrum are developing software systems that transform two-dimensional CT or MRI images into three-dimensional views of the individual patient's anatomy. These 3D-images, which can be turned in any direction, help surgeons to precisely plan the upcoming surgical intervention. Thus, they can assess whether the tumor is locally restricted or has already grown into neighboring tissues. The three-dimensional views also show which tissue areas might be cut off from blood supply as a result of the surgery. This enables one to recognize and minimize complications in advance. Moreover, the software also provides quantitative information about organ volumes and safety distances around high-risk organs which are not directly recognizable from the original two-dimensional data. The 3D-images are also available during surgery via a monitor.

Spatial orientation will be easier for surgeons who have prepared for an intervention using the 3D-images. Thus, they can operate in a shorter time – which benefits the patient. This is the expectation of Professor Hans-Peter Meinzer, head of the Division of Medical and Biological Informatics.

The software system, which is already established in liver surgery at the University Surgical Hospital in Heidelberg, was first tested in pancreatic surgery in 2005. The doctors and computer scientists involved are currently conducting a study to find out whether the use of the software measurably improves surgery results.

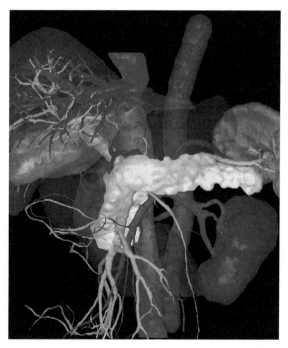

Three-dimensional representation of the pancreas (yellow). Vital large blood vessels are located in the immediate vicinity

Therefore, a catheter, pushed through the arteries to the pancreas, served as a transport vehicle. Thus, the capsule are delivered to their destination safely and directly. Ifosfamide is subsequently administered systemically, although at much lower dosages than previously. Since the chemotherapy drug is now metabolized directly in the pancreas, its efficacy has improved while dosage of the substance has decreased.

The treatment principle proved to be successful: In two of 14 patients participating in the study the tumor in the pancreas shrunk. In eleven more patients at least the state of health stabilized. Of the patients treated by the new method, three times as many survived the first year than of those study participants who had received the standard chemotherapy, gemcitabine. "We can take this as a first positive result", concludes Löhr, "but our declared goal is to completely eliminate the tumors through the treatment or at least shrink them to a size allowing surgical removal."

Catheters as Drug Delivery Highways

In the meantime, Löhr and his team have also tested the capsule method in patients. Phase I and II clinical trials have been completed. First, another hurdle had to be overcome. Direct injection of the capsules is not an option for humans, because the pancreas is hidden too deep within the body and the risk of injuring an organ with the injection needle would be too high.

For this reason, the researchers of the Clinical Cooperation Unit "Molecular Gastroenterology" are currently pursuing new clinical research projects to investigate how the combination of gene therapy and chemotherapy may be further improved. To this end, they are experimenting with improved gene constructs containing genes for alternative metabolic enzymes. Another approach under study are substances known as enhancers, which boost gene expression. The re-

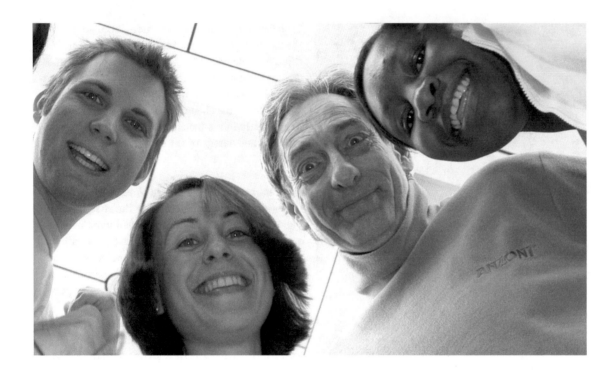

searchers hope that all this taken together will eventually further enhance ifosfamide metabolization. In addition, Löhr's research team is working to improve the capsules to make them last longer and thus extend their service in the sick pancreas.

New Fields of Application

The combination of gene therapy and chemotherapy is suitable not only for the treatment of pancreatic cancer. In first promising experiments with laboratory mice, Löhr's team has successfully tested this therapy method to treat malignant ascites – a condition in which fluid collects in the abdomen as a result of cancer of the peritoneum. The therapeutic capsules containing the genetically engineered cells were injected here together with ifosfamide directly into the abdominal cavity where they metabolized the drug. In the animal model, the treatment was effective for abdominal cancers, too. The tumors shrunk significantly in all mice.

Soon this treatment approach will be tested in clinical trials. Studies are scheduled for the second half of 2006 in which the scientists want to find out whether the new mode of treating malignant ascites is also promising in humans. If it stands the trial, the drug

that was almost discarded would not only have made a comeback, it could even open up new avenues – in combination with Löhr's capsules – for treating further cancers that are difficult to treat.

Stefanie Reinberger

Literature

Samel, S. et al., Cancer Gene Therapy 13:65, 2006
Löhr, M. et al., Cancer Therapy 1:121, 2003
Löhr, M. et al., Lancet 357:1591, 2001

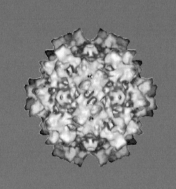

Research Program
Infection and Cancer

Viruses play a crucial role in a number of cancers. Several divisions of this Research Program investigate the mechanisms by which viruses cause cancer and develop and test vaccines that help the body to fight off such infections. In addition, researchers are isolating and characterizing unknown viruses from tumor material.

Parvoviruses are capable of specifically killing cancer cells. Scientists are attempting to use this property to develop a new therapeutic approach to cancers that are difficult to treat, such as glioblastoma. Furthermore, they are testing various viruses as vehicles for introducing therapeutic genes into cells.

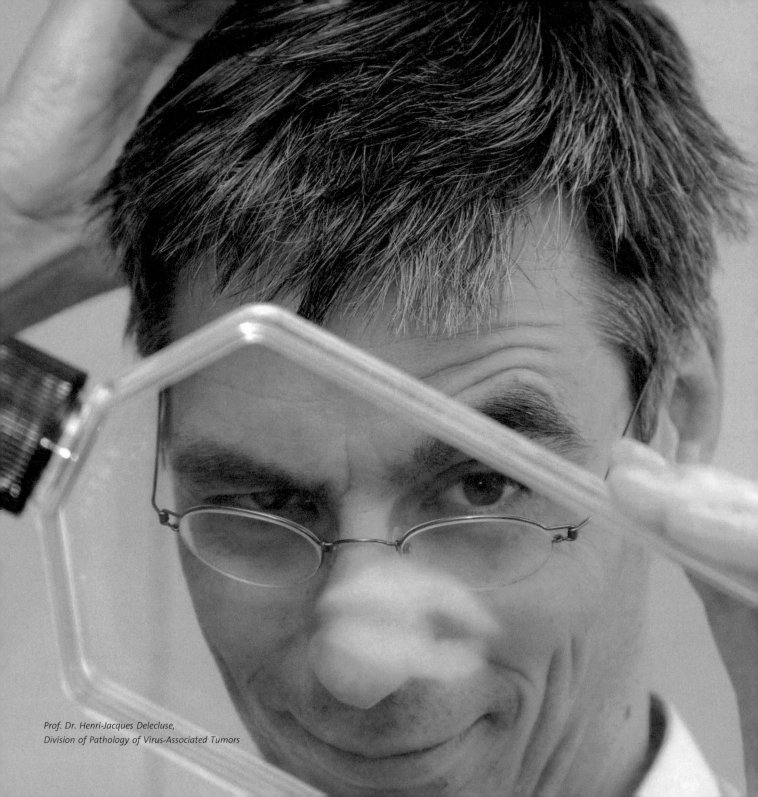

Prof. Dr. Henri-Jacques Delecluse,
Division of Pathology of Virus-Associated Tumors

From Infection to Cancer: Catching the Virus in the Act

The Epstein-Barr virus causes kissing disease and is highly suspected to be responsible for the development of a number of cancers

The year was 1911. Francis Peyton Rous, a young scientist working at the New York Rockefeller Institute, came up with a theory that seemed almost unbelievable. He postulated that viruses cause cancer. In a spectacular experiment he had been able to transmit tumors from sick chicken to healthy birds. At the time, Rous was little acknowledged by the scientific community which ridiculed his observation as a curiosity with little or no potential relevance for mankind. Far from it! Over the years, it became increasingly clear that even more virus types can cause cancer, even in humans. Rous was awarded the Nobel Prize in 1966.

Today, scientists believe that viruses are causally involved in 15 to 20 percent of cancer cases. Some experts estimate this number to be even higher. The list of suspected viruses is long: It includes hepatitis viruses as well as a number of papillomaviruses and herpesviruses, to name just a few examples. But things are not as simple and clear in humans as they were in Rous' chickens. Human tumor viruses seem to cause cancer only under very specific conditions – and most of these have not yet been sufficiently studied.

Professor Henri-Jacques Delecluse, head of the Division of Pathogenesis of Virus-Associated Tumors at the DKFZ, has set out to change this – at least as far as a virus called Epstein-Barr virus (EBV) is concerned. This member of the herpesvirus family is particularly mysterious and is unknown to most people. Yet about 95 percent of the population are infected by this virus – about as many as by its most famous relative, the herpes simplex virus that causes painful lip blisters with unpleasant regularity in some people.

From "Kissing Disease" to Cancer

When EBV infection occurs during childhood, it usually causes no symptoms. During adolescence or adulthood it often causes infectious mononucleosis, a disease with symptoms including fever, sore throat, and swollen lymph glands. Due to its transmission via infected saliva it is also called "kissing disease".

But no matter what happens at primary infection, the virus inevitably leaves its footprints: Its genome re-

mains in the nucleus of infected cells like an additional chromosome. In infected persons with no symptoms, about one in 10,000 B cells – a specific type of
white blood cells of the immune system (see box on
page 104) – is host to the viral genetic information. It
generally remains unnoticed but can become active
under certain conditions such as immunosuppression
in recipients of organ transplants or in AIDS patients,
but also for other, yet unknown reasons. The consequences are fatal: Reactivated (secondary) EBV infections cause various cancers including B cell lymphomas such as Burkitt's lymphoma and Hodgkin's disease. Also known are pathologically transformed T
cells as well as transformed epithelial cells in the na-
sopharynx. The virus is also found in five to ten percent of gastric carcinoma cases. The incidences of the
different EBV-associated tumor diseases are character-
istically increased in different regions: Hodgkin's disease in Europe, T cell lymphoma in Japan, Burkitt's
lymphoma in Africa and a type of nasopharyngeal
carcinoma in Northern Africa.

This extraordinary variety of different diseases makes
it no easier for researchers to define the causes and
mechanisms that lead to EBV-associated tumors. "Another problem is that although the WHO has long
since defined EBV as a tumor virus, we have hardly
any hard proof that it is really responsible for cancer
development", explains Delecluse, adding: "The fact
that we find viruses in the transformed cells is not
sufficient to prove the carcinogenic properties of such
a common virus." Only in the case of patients who de-

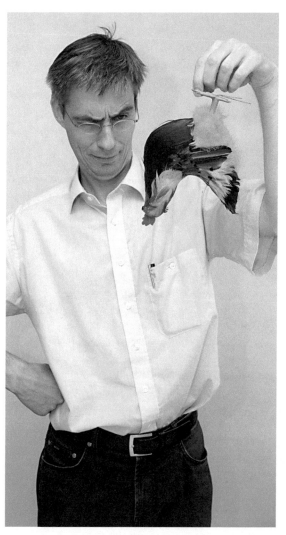

velop a condition called posttransplant lymphoproliferative disorder, or PTLD for short, scientists have been able to prove that EBV causes this cancer.

Wanted: A Cell Culture System for Infection Experiments

So far, the limiting factor for research efforts has been the lack of a cell culture system. In order to study the disease-causing mechanisms of a virus, infection experiments in the culture dish are indispensable. But these turned out to be a great problem in the case of EBV: Although researchers worldwide are working with EBV-infected cell lines, these tissue cultures are only of limited usefulness when it comes to proving tumorigenic processes.

When the virus is added to B lymphocytes in a culture bottle, a typical transformation of the cells is observed. They start to proliferate heavily and become immortal. A closer look at the virus in the B cells shows that the tissue cultures reflect the exact situation that occurs in transplant recipients with PTLD. In these cases the virus expresses the same genes as in the culture bottle. But this also means that EBV-immortalized B lymphocytes give no clues about the development of other B cell lymphomas such as Burkitt's lymphoma or Hodgkin's disease. For in these cases only a fraction of the more than one hundred viral genes are active, significantly less than in PTLD.

A Dream Within Reach

If viruses can cause cancer, then an appropriate vaccine should protect against these tumor diseases. What sounded like wishful thinking for a long time has in fact become reality now. In summer 2006 the US Food and Drug Administration has approved a vaccine against human papillomaviruses (wart viruses, HPV). The vaccine protects women against cervical cancer, the dangerous late effect of an infection with this virus.

Scientists of the Deutsches Krebsforschungszentrum contributed a great deal to the finding that there is a connection between seemingly harmless wart viruses and cervical cancer. Most often wart viruses cause benign lesions in the skin or mucous membranes. However, certain members of this virus group, in particular HPV16 and HPV18, cause cervical cancer in some infected women. Former Scientific Director Professor Harald zur Hausen, jointly with Professor Lutz Gissmann – who today leads the Division of Genome Alterations and Carcinogenesis – were able to isolate and characterize HPV16 and HPV18 from tumor material. Today it is known that tissue samples from 99.7 percent of cervical cancer patients contain papillomaviruses. Gissmann and his co-workers later developed methods for efficient production of what are called virus-like particles (VLPs). VLPs are empty protein shells of the virus that contain no genetic material, which makes them a safe vaccine.

The vaccine, which will probably be launched at the German market already in 2006, is directed against the main cancer causing virus types HPV16 and 18 and also against HPV6 and 11 that cause genital warts. It protects against about 70 percent of cervical cancers. In clinical trials including 25,000 women it was found to prevent precancerous lesions associated with HPV16 or HPV18 to one hundred percent.

In the meantime, the Heidelberg virologists are already working on a second-generation vaccine: small pellets called capsomeres that are composed of just five units of the L1 viral protein. Capsomeres are much easier and cheaper to produce than the virus-like particles used so far, while prodding an equally effective immune reaction. In addition, DKFZ researchers are developing methods for administering the vaccine by inhalation rather than by injection. To this end, they use adeno-associated viruses as gene ferries to introduce the genetic information for specific viral proteins into an organism. First studies with mice have shown that this can bring about long-lasting immunity against papillomaviruses.

Things are even more complicated with T lymphocytes and epithelial cells. For many years researchers have not been able to even infect these cells with the virus – at least not with those viral strains that are normally used in the lab. Possibly, the laboratory variants of EBV are adjusted to conditions in B cell cultures so much that they are no longer able to infect other cell types. But experiments using viruses obtained directly from patients have also failed so far. This suggests that the culture conditions or the cells themselves – quite possible for the manifold epithelial tissues – might also not be ideal. "Moreover, isolated viruses multiply extremely slowly even in B cells", says Delecluse. With a smile he continues: "Sometimes you could think EBV has forgotten that it is a virus and has to proliferate."

A Protein Is Key to Success

Working with laboratory strains and viruses isolated from patients the researcher noticed a difference between them. Commonly used laboratory viruses distinguish themselves from their "wild-type" relatives on the surface in one particular protein molecule named gp110 (glycoprotein 110) that contains sugar molecules. It is found much less in viruses adjusted to the conditions in the culture bottle. "At present we still don't know for sure what the function of this protein is, but there is reason to believe that it plays a role in docking at and invading the host cell", Delecluse says explaining the relevance of this molecule.

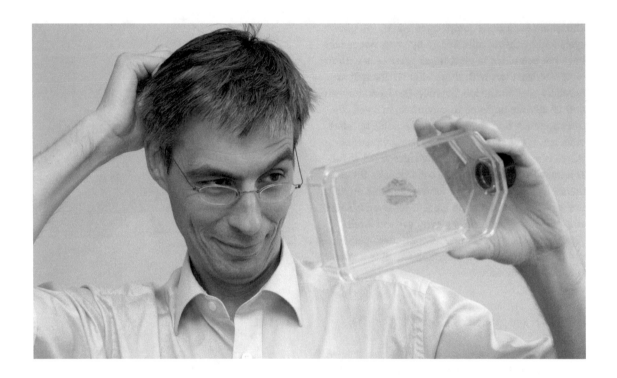

This observation indicates that laboratory viruses in a culture dish fail to proliferate due to their lack of gp110 in epithelial or T cells. Thus, Delecluse and his co-worker Bernhard Neuhierl, together with a research group headed by veterinary researcher Wolfgang Hammerschmidt in Munich, came up with an idea: If it were possible to increase the amount of the surface protein, the virus should be better able to infect cells. The scientists therefore introduced the genetic infor-

mation for gp110 into an infected B cell line. There the viral protein would be formed and give rise to a new, more infectious virus generation.

The concept proved to be right. Stimulation of these manipulated and EBV infected cells gave rise to a new virus generation – with a significantly higher proportion of gp110 on their surface. As subsequent experiments showed, these "spiced up" viruses not only have a much better ability to infect B cell lines, they were even capable of infecting epithelial cells. Thus, Delecluse and his colleagues have developed the first EBV culture system that can be used for studying other cell types than B lymphocytes. Moreover, this finally provides scientists with a tool for closely studying the pathogen's life cycle and cancer-causing mechanisms – at least in epithelial cells.

The researchers in Delecluse's Division at the Deutsches Krebsforschungszentrum are taking a closer look at gp110 and its role in infection. They have already established that the surface molecule is absolutely vital for infecting epithelial cells. Analyzing the gene coding for this glycoprotein is also of great importance. For the individual virus strains often show differences in their gp110 molecules – and this is where we might find the answer to the question why

the virus is able to infect different cell types and cause such diverse cancer types. And why EBV-associated tumors are found in such varying incidences and types depending on the geographical region.

"The great goal, however, is to gather sufficient information about the virus to enable us to eventually develop a vaccine", says Delecluse, adding emphatically: "But to achieve this we have to make the public aware of EBV and its threats and thus make vaccine research a more urgent case."

Stefanie Reinberger

Literature

Neuhierl, B. et al.: PNAS 99:15036, 2002
Timms, J. M. et al.: Lancet 361:217, 2003

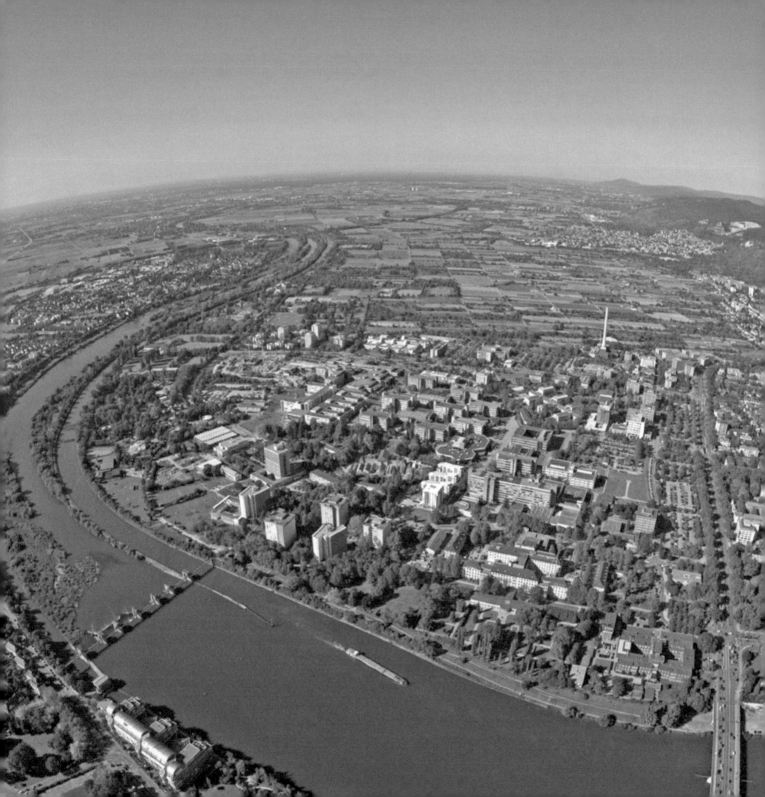

The NCT Heidelberg: A Joint Venture against Cancer

"Right now we still have to manage with 18 treatment spaces. But in the new building we expect to deliver about 150 outpatient chemotherapy treatments daily," says PD Dr. Dirk Jäger, describing the planned capacities of the outpatient clinic of the National Center for Tumor Diseases (NCT) Heidelberg. Construction of the new building in the Neuenheimer Feld is scheduled to start in 2006. Until the new building is completed, the NCT is temporarily housed in the Otto Meyerhof Center of the University Hospitals. Dirk Jäger has been head of the area "Medical Oncology" since July 2005. Since the NCT was established, most of the specialty hospitals working in oncology in Heidelberg have set up oncological consulting hours at the Meyerhof Center. This system of outpatient units connected to the

hospitals is the core activity of the interdisciplinary Tumor Outpatient Unit, which is a central point of reference open to all cancer patients in Heidelberg. "Unlike in the past, cancer patients in Heidelberg are no longer referred to a specific hospital, but to the interdisciplinary Tumor Outpatient Unit, which operates as a portal to the NCT," Jäger explains. "Currently, most of our patients come from this region. But we have noticed that we are also becoming increasingly attractive for sufferers from outside the region who seek a second or third opinion. For example, many patients with pancreatic cancer come here, because the expertise of Heidelberg surgeons in this field is acknowledged nationally and internationally."

The NCT was established by the Heidelberg University Hospitals, the Medical Faculty of Heidelberg University, the Heidelberg Thorax Clinic, and the Deutsches Krebsforschungszen-

trum (German Cancer Research Center, DKFZ) and modeled after the U.S. Comprehensive Cancer Centers. Quality-assured, interdisciplinary patient care are substantial requirements of this concept; another characteristic feature of the U.S. example is a close connection of clinical practice and clinical cancer research under one roof.

The DKFZ contributes chiefly the scientific part of the NCT: The clinical area "Medical Oncology" is supplemented by the two clinical-scientific research areas "Translational Oncology" and "Preventive Oncology". Professor Dr. Christof von Kalle, director of the NCT and head of the Translational Oncology division since July 2005, describes the opportunities arising for both sides from the close collaboration between clinical research and patient care: "Our goal is to offer participation in clinical trials at the NCT to as many patients as possible so that they can benefit from innovative methods

PD Dr. Dirk Jäger (left), head of the Clinical Oncology Division and Prof. Christof von Kalle, head of the NCT Heidelberg and the Translational Oncology Division

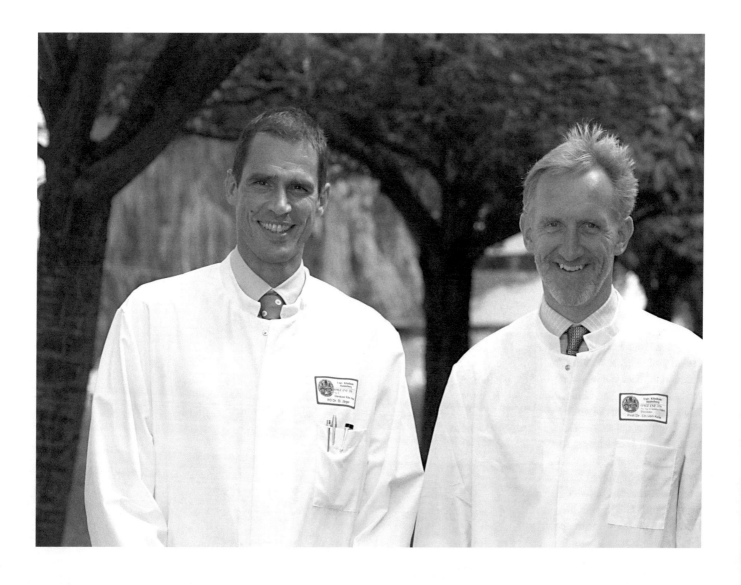

and the latest and best medical care. This will often be investigator initiated trials, in which substances or methods developed at Heidelberg research institutes are tested in early-stage clinical trials. On the other hand, with an estimated number of patients of up to 8,000 per year, we are also an interesting partner for large-scale approval trials for new drugs from the pharmaceutical industry."

To systematically get clinical trials to the NCT, the concept provides for a Clinical Trials Center, which advises doctors and researchers in the complex design and helps to include patients who meet the relevant inclusion criteria. The Clinical Trials Center is part of an infrastructure that makes the NCT attractive for translational research projects: All patient data are filed in anonymized form in a centralized clinical cancer register, thus creating an invaluable data resource for epidemiological studies. In addi-

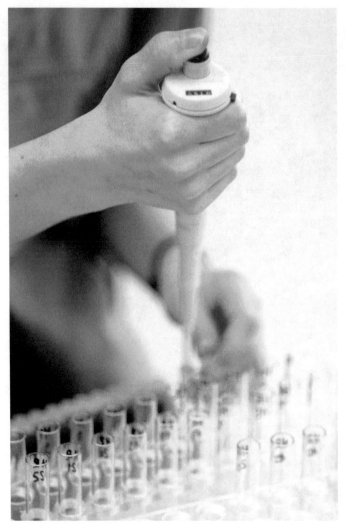

tion, scientists will have access to a central image database as well as a tumor and serum bank.

Research for the Patient

Alongside von Kalle's division, the area "Translational Oncology" comprises the seven Clinical Cooperation Units and further clinically oriented research groups of the DKFZ. The common goal of all projects assigned to this area can be summarized as follows: To improve the effectiveness of treatment methods, particularly for those cancers where medics can hardly do anything yet, to direct them more specifically

against cancer cells and make them gentler for the body, thus improving the patients' quality of life. Von Kalle plans to investigate in his division which marker molecules are characteristic of cancer stem cells, which are the basis of uncontrolled growth of malignant tumors. Thus he aims to identify new target structures for treatments against the most dangerous cells of a tumor. In addition, researchers in his division are working on methods to improve protection of bone marrow cells against the toxic effect of chemotherapy drugs so that patients may be treated with higher, and thus more effective, drug doses.

DKFZ researchers are planning to test, within the framework of the NCT, the effectiveness of an antibody for treating tumor-associated pleural effusion and are designing a phase II trial of an immune therapy using activated memory T cells from the bone marrow of patients with advanced breast cancer.

Some tumor diseases – such as pancreatic cancer, in many cases – are associated with a condition called cachexia, a severe form of wasting, which usually goes along with an unfavorable disease progression. A study planned at the NCT is aimed at identifying factors causing the severe weight loss and intervene by a special diet, exercise and drugs.

For the Helmholtz Association of National Research Centers, of which the DKFZ is a member, the transfer of results from basic research into clinical application is a major goal. By providing funds of about 12 million euros, the science organization recog-

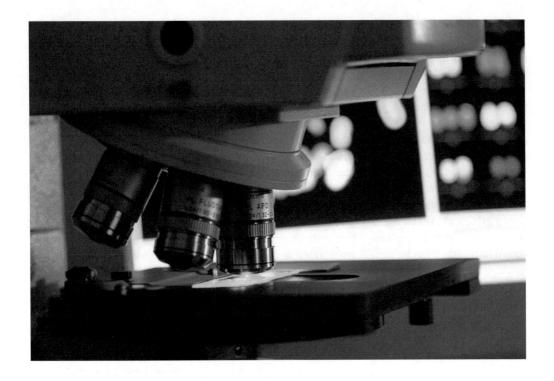

nizes the NCT's consistent attention to translational research projects. The Heidelberg project receives additional support from the Deutsche Krebshilfe (German Cancer Aid), which will prefinance the new building of the NCT.

The goal of the second NCT research area, "Preventive Oncology", is to prevent cancer or to stop the disease process at an early stage. The three DKFZ divisions, "Clinical Epidemiology", "Molecular-Genetic Epidemiology", and "Toxicology and Cancer Risk Factors", are assigned to

this area. Cancer prevention has become increasingly important in oncology in recent years. Efforts include testing of substances with cancer preventing properties, development of innovative screening methods for the detection of precancerous lesions, designing new concepts of primary and secondary cancer prevention as well as identifying genetic and environmental factors which increase the individual cancer risk.

Institutionalized Transparency

For patients who come to the central Tumor Outpatient Unit, a cancer diagnosis has usually been established. At the NCT, they will be examined and their data will be documented in an electronic patient record. An interdisciplinary general or specialized tumor board discusses unclear cases on the day

of a patient's presentation and jointly issues a treatment recommendation. Thus it is guaranteed that no patient will go home without a result. Patients will then receive further treatment in the Heidelberg University specialty hospitals; all outpatient chemotherapy treatments are conducted centrally at the NCT's outpatient clinic.

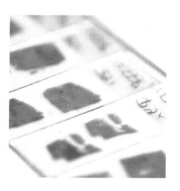

Treatment recommendations follow the NCT's own treatment guidelines. These Standard Operating Procedures (SOPs) are developed for each tumor entity by an expert panel comprising doctors of different disciplines as well as experts from research, care and counseling services.

The third pillar of the NCT, alongside treatment and research, is patient education and information. Linked to the Tumor Outpatient Unit is a comprehensive range of services including dietary and human genetic counseling, support of smoking cessation, psychoso-

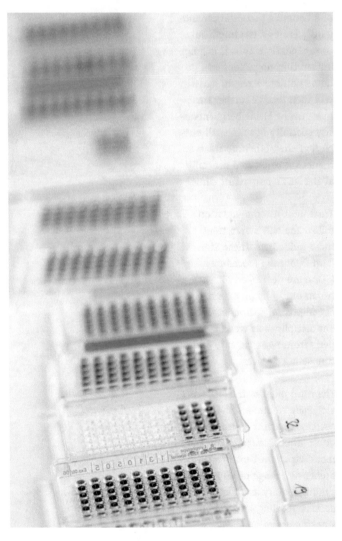

cial care and clinical social services. The DKFZ's Cancer Information Service, KID, which is normally available only by phone or email, has set up a regular counseling service at the NCT. "People are often asking about the so-called unconventional treatment methods, about dietary supplements and strengthening of the immune system," says Dr. Ingeborg Traut, who represents KID at the NCT twice weekly. "Many patients wish to make their own contribution to healing in addition to a conventional medical treatment." The direct personal encounters during appointments at the NCT were something new for KID staff member Traut. "Here I experience the fears and concerns of the advice-seekers much more directly than at the other end of the telephone line," Traut explains. "The advantage for our patients is that they find competent contact persons at the various counseling services, right here and now, for all their questions, be it about a treatment recommendation, a necessary change of diet or cost coverage by the health insurance."

"The times when it was either surgery or radiotherapy are long gone. Treatment options for cancer today are so complex that some institution with a bridging function is needed to coordinate, on the one hand, the different clinical disciplines and to make sure, on the other hand, that innovative treatment concepts make their way to the patients," says Dirk Jäger. "To this end, the Heidelberg NCT has developed an exciting and convincing concept; here we pursue modern oncology according to disclosed standard guidelines with consistent transparency. There is no other place yet where this is institutionalized in this form. With the NCT, we strive to achieve a standard in Germany that has been normal in the U.S. for many years."

Sibylle Kohlstädt

Down-to-Earth Measures to Protect Highly Inspired Ideas

Like the ranges and valleys of a mountain massif on a relief map, the spatial structure of methyltransferase is shown in a three-dimensional representation on the computer screen. In a kind of virtual jigsaw puzzle, researchers are able to dock small molecules to the enzyme until they fit like a key in a lock. Frank Lyko was searching for a key to block this lock.

The fitting molecule was eventually found in a substance database of the US National Cancer Research Institute. Lyko's collaboration partners of the Division of Molecular Toxicology at the German Cancer Research Center were able to produce the substance synthetically. The big moment came when first tests showed that RG108 – as the key molecule is called – holds in the test tube what it had promised on the

screen: By binding to the active center of methyltransferase, the substance appears to block the enzyme's activity.

Methyltransferases have been in the focus of cancer medicine for years. Scientists expect that it may be possible to reprogram tumor cells into normal cells using specific inhibitors of these enzymes (see box on page 163). From the start, Dr. Frank Lyko, head of the Division of Epigenetics, was aware that he may have found a real treasure in RG108 – both from the medical and economic perspectives. Almost all big pharmaceutical companies had been searching for similarly acting substances. High time for Lyko to secure the rights to the sought-after substance.

Publication Prohibited for the Time Being

According the German Employee Invention Act, scientists are obliged to report to their employer any invention that arises from their work. To do so, researchers at the DKFZ are requested to contact the Office of Technology Transfer, which will accompany them on the long road leading from an invention over patenting to commercial exploitation of the invention and marketing of a potential product. First contact between researchers and technology managers is usually established through an invention disclosure. Using the answers provided by the inventor in this form, the technology transfer staff can clarify the essentials right away: Is the invention novel or has it already been published in any form? Researchers are questioned whether they might already have disclosed details of the imminent scientific breakthrough in a conversation with

This could be a treasure: Dr. Frank Lyko (left) presents his invention for the first time to Dr. Christian Kliem of the Technology Transfer Division

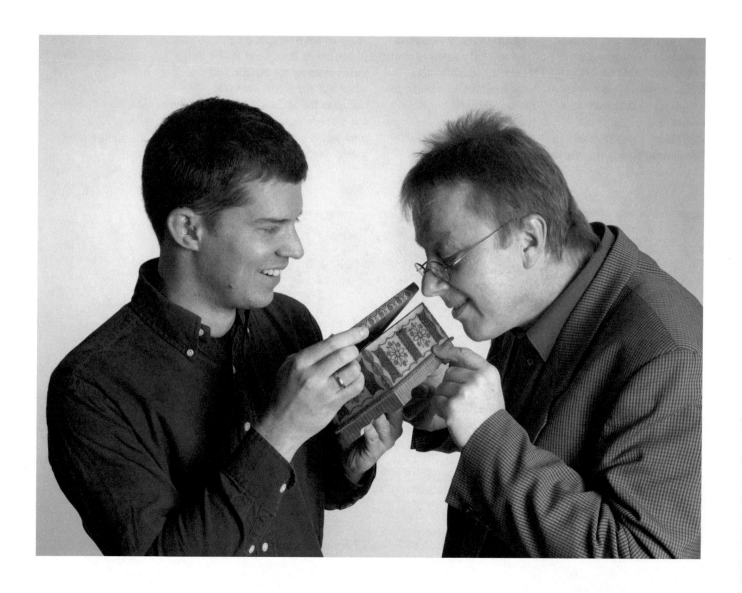

colleagues at the last specialist conference. For a patent application, this would be, in legal terms, "prejudicial to novelty". If a patent application is considered, it is crucial that it is filed before any publication. In this process, researchers rely on the cooperation of all parties involves. In the case of doctoral theses, the assessors may even agree to silence in advance and the deanship will keep the printed copies of the thesis under lock and key until the application is filed.

The relevant date according to patent law is the date of publication of an article, not the date when the manuscript was submitted to the journal. Considering that several months usually pass between the two dates, a patent application does not

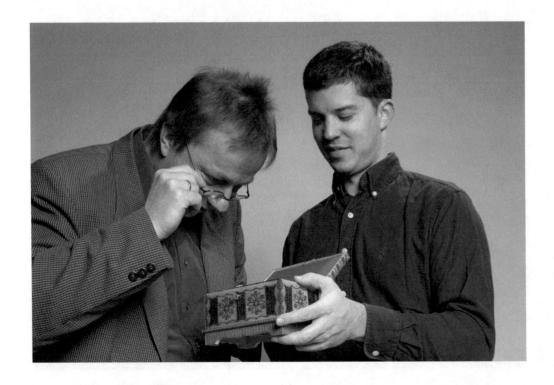

Methyl Silences Genes

Nature has provided for a special kind of labeling for genes whose activity is to be reduced: Specialized enzymes called methyltransferases attach small hydrocarbon compounds (methyl groups) to specific sites of the DNA. Only the cytosine in a base sequence of cytosine-guanosine (CG) gets labeled with a methyl group. In the human genome, such CG pairs are underrepresented. However, they accumulate in what are called promoter areas that serve as on/off switches for genes. In healthy cells, these sequences are usually present in an unmethylated state. A typical characteristic of almost all tumors, however, is an overmethylation of the promoter areas. As a result, the switches are set in "off" position so that many important genes cease to function. If this includes genes that slow down the cell cycle, then uncontrolled cell growth may be the consequence. Or worse, if genes are silenced that are responsible for repairing defects in the genetic material, then the floodgates are open to further mutations.

Such "epigenetic" mutations as methylation are reversible. The cell uses these to regulate gene activity and it can selectively introduce and remove them. The methyl labels have to be newly placed with every cell division cycle. This is where scientists try to intervene and reprogram tumor cells into normal cells. Their goal is to selectively switch off the enzymes that are responsible for methylation. A first inhibitor of methyltransferase was found in 5-azacytidin. However, like other related substances, the compound needs to be integrated into the genome, which is toxic for the cells.

Using computer-assisted modeling of human DNA methyltransferase, a research team in Frank Lyko's division at the Deutsches Krebsforschungszentrum was able to identify a low-molecular inhibitor of the enzyme. The substance called RG108 acts through direct binding to the transferase. Experiments in the culture dish demonstrate that RG108 significantly reduces methylation without damaging the cells.

normally delay publication. For online publications, this time span is much shorter so that it can get tight sometimes. Therefore, the technology transfer staff advises scientists to contact them as early as possible.

The second important question already requires a great deal of expertise in patent law matters: Is the invention really an invention or, possibly, only a discovery? "An invention must solve a problem", explains Dr. Ruth Herzog, head of the Division of Technology Transfer. "There is a mnemonic that helps to distinguish between the two: A discovery is an increment to knowledge, an invention to skills." A third criterion is the capability of industrial application. While this ranges third in patent law, it is crucial for the Technology Transfer Office: "We only invest in patent applications if we are convinced of the commercial exploitation potential of an invention. In the case of RG108,

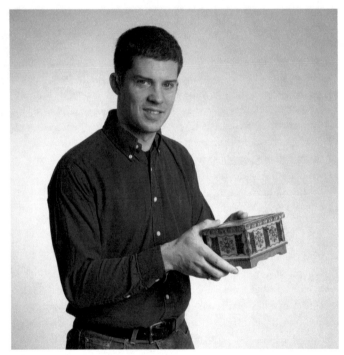

there was no doubt about this", says Herzog.

New Working Principle with High Potential

Having received the invention disclosure by Lyko and co-workers, the technology transfer staff went about evaluating the patentability of the invention. This involves extensive searches in the specialist literature and patent databases. In addition, the technology transfer managers conduct market research in order to assess the

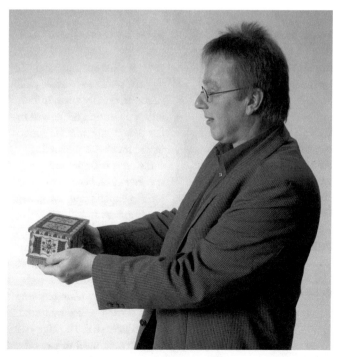

commercial value of the invention. If the patent experts come to the conclusion that there are no formal or subject-matter impediments to patenting the invention and that it also has good economic potential, then Technology Transfer will recommend pursuit of patenting the invention to the Management Board of the DKFZ and will simultaneously propose a filing strategy.

If the Board follows the recommendations, the German Cancer Research Center thus claims the employee invention. If not, inventors are free to exploit their invention on their own initiative and at their own expense.

In the case of RG108, the technology transfer managers agreed that this is an invention of a new working principle of an anticancer drug with high economic potential. Jointly with the researchers, an external patent attorney then drafted the patent specification.

To do so, it is not enough to simply jot down the structural formula of RG108. "This would make it easy for competitors", says technology transfer team member Dr. Christian Kliem, who used to work as a chemist at the DKFZ. "Exchanging a seemingly unimportant side chain of our molecule would be sufficient to circumvent our patent." Chemical laypersons will hardly recognize R108 from the formula that is eventually submitted to the patent office. Every single functional group, every single side chain of the compound is defined as broadly as possible. By doing so, the applicants are trying to include in the patent protection every possible variant of RG108 that might also act as an inhibitor of methyltransferase. Alongside a description of the production and purification of the substance, the patent specification contains what are called patent "claims": For

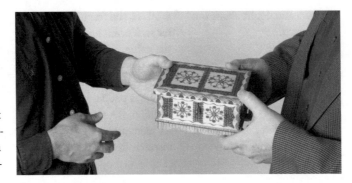

RG108, these comprise the production and any conceivable use of the substance in the treatment of any cancer disease.

Over six months have elapsed between the invention disclosure and the filing of the patent application for RG108 at the European Patent Office. The Office's task is now to find out whether documents and publications exist that may be opposed to the patent or the claims in their desired scope, respectively.

The Effort Should Pay Off

From the date of the patent filing, the road to scientific publication is usually open. In fact, once publication is allowed under patent law, it is very much in the interest of technology transfer: It is important that the invention becomes known among experts and that potential licensees from the pharmaceutical industry take notice of the new substance. While the application is being examined at the patent office, the technology transfer team has long since started searching for potential licensees. The high costs of patenting need to pay off as soon as possible. At this time, RG108 is still at a very early stage of product development. The substance first has to pass numerous preclinical tests before it can be used in clinical trials. Although the German Cancer Research Center has plans to become more actively involved in this stage of drug development in the future and, thus, to close the gap between medical fundamental research and clinical research, the costs of further developing a substance at present exceed the research institute's financial possibilities by far. Therefore, the ideal license candidate would be a company that advances the substance through the various stages of preclinical and clinical testing. In return for the rights to RG108, the company would have to pay license fees to the DKFZ – in the form of down payments, milestone payments, and running license royalties if a product is eventually sold.

In the case of RG108, the pharmaceutical industry showed a great deal of interest. However, the companies rated the entry risk as too high because the invention is yet too little developed. But the technology managers have found a collaboration partner for Lyko: Cancer Research UK, the UK equivalent to the German Cancer Aid (Deutsche Krebshilfe), has founded its own technology transfer company named Cancer Research Technology Limited (CRT). One of the goals of CRT is to find commercial partners for possibly swift development of important results in cancer research – so that cancer patients may benefit as soon as possible from innovative therapeutics.

A compensation deal was reached with CRT: Cancer Research UK will provide personnel and material support for Lyko's research. At the same time, CRT is granted the license rights to RG108 and will start preclinical studies. In addition,

the UK partner will try to synthesize new, possibly even more effective variants of RG108, which Frank Lyko will test in his cellular test systems. If CRT finds a commercial partner who agrees to take on the further development of RG108, then the DKFZ and CRT will divide license revenues according to a special ratio. In addition, CRT will also have variants of RG108 produced which are not covered by the patent. Should a licensee be found for one of these substances, the division of revenues will change.

The Pitfalls of the License Agreement

What sounds simple was a tough job in practice. The drafting of a license agreement, which must be tailored to the interests of both partners, is a task for experts and may take several months. For the DKFZ, there are not only economic, but also scientific interests involved. Thus, it is crucial to en-

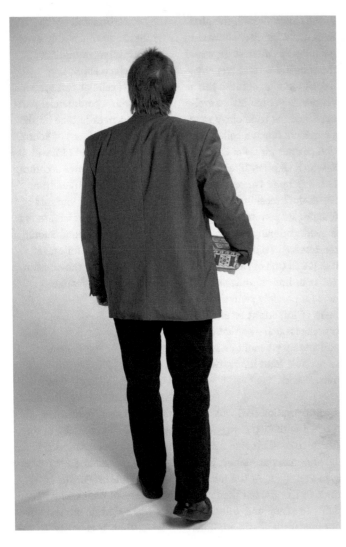

sure that Frank Lyko does not lose the rights to his own research by signing the agreement. It is important, for example, that it is still allowed for the scientist to collaborate in the licensed area with other companies – also for commercial purposes. Different stipulations may well lead to an isolated position of the scientist. "We try to make sure that companies actually use the licenses and exploit the invention", Herzog and Kliem explain. Otherwise, a promising approach in cancer treatment might be blocked for several years. Appropriate additional clauses in the licensing agreement – such as defined milestones and a right to terminate the agreement – serve to safeguard these arrangements.

Kliem's task in these negotiations is to evaluate the economic aspects and to take account of the inventor's scientific interests. It is the task of lawyer Peter Piesche to wrap all terms agreed upon into legally waterproof clauses. Piesche specializes in elaborating the wording of complex legal contracts.

"We are convinced that CRT will help us to obtain new data about the effectiveness of RG108 and thus to attract a pharmaceutical company for further clinical development.

A more advanced development stage reduces the entry risk for the company – even though it has to pay a higher price then."

Frank Lyko is currently studying derivatives of RG108 for improved effectiveness. He is sure that his mental "baby" is in good hands with CRT. "I never wanted to conduct research only in the ivory tower. It was always important to me that it eventually all leads to something that helps patients." Thus, jointly with Technology Transfer, the scientist will follow with anticipation and curiosity the progress of his idea along its long road to a product.

Sibylle Kohlstädt

The International PhD-Program – Mutual Benefits

Thursday morning at 9 am: Time for a further lecture in the series 'Progress in Cancer Research', a required course for all doctoral students at the Ger-man Cancer Research Center. From apoptosis to the cyclotron – over the course of six semesters, internal experts cover the entire spectrum of the Center's scientific activities. At the end of this period, the course begins anew. "In this way we can be sure that every PhD student, over the duration of their three-year doctoral work, has the opportunity to learn about the full range of our research", explains PD Dr. Thomas Efferth, coordinator of the International PhD Program of the German Cancer Research Center.

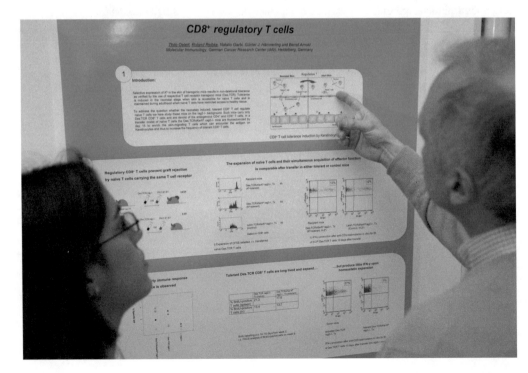

Maria Papatriantafyllou from Athens was able to convince the selection commission. Since 2005, she has been performing research as a PhD student at the DKFZ

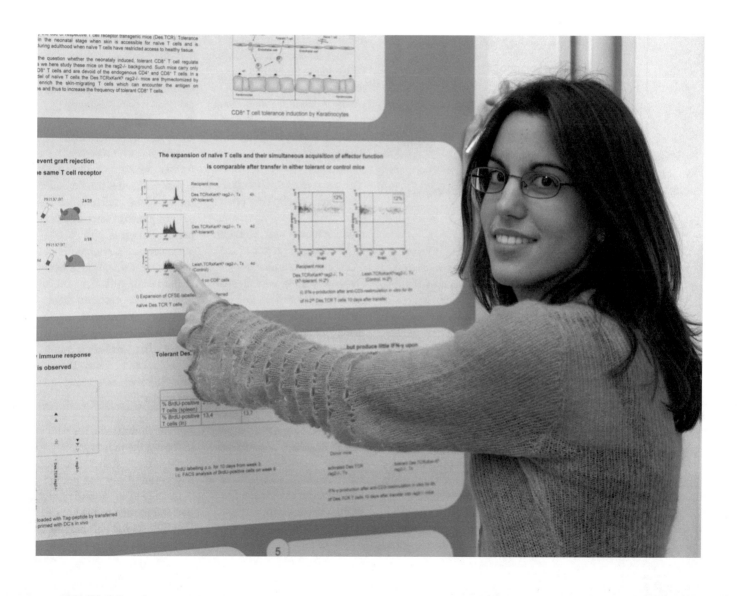

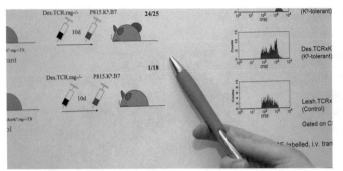

The lecture course is just one part of the extensive further education provided by the DKFZ for the coming generation of scientists. Seminars and courses in presentation skills and scientific English are as much a part of the scheme as workshops on laboratory methods. Participation is not entirely voluntary: For every teaching event students receive 'credit points', of which everyone has to have collected 15 by the end of their doctoral course. Points are also awarded for giving presentations of scientific results at congresses, at the internal DKFZ poster competition,

and at the annual weekend seminar for doctoral students. To stimulate interest in complementary activities, attendance at public relations events and participation in social activities are also rewarded with credit points.

"For me, it is more a motivation than a compulsory program", says Maria Papatriantafyllou, who has been working on her doctoral project at the DKFZ since September 2005. The young Greek woman studied biology in Athens and developed an interest in immunology while working on her diploma. Seeking a suitable place to do a PhD, her extensive Internet researches led her by chance to discover the PhD program of the German Cancer Research Center. After her professors in Athens had assured her that the DKFZ is one of Europe's foremost addresses for immunology, she sent in her written application.

Three Selection Processes per Year

Of the roughly 400 applicants per year, a commission of about 15 internal scientists – group and divisional heads – selects the best 20 percent for a further evaluation. Three times a year candidates from all over the world are invited to Heidelberg to present themselves in person. Here they must convince the commission with an eight-minute scientific presentation and an interview. On each of these occasions, there are roughly 12 successful candidates, who then find themselves in the enviable position of being able to choose their future division or working group at will.

Even applicants who are not chosen at the presentation stage, often find that their journey to Heidelberg was not in vain: Only about a third of all doctoral positions are allocated centrally via the PhD program, the remaining larger number

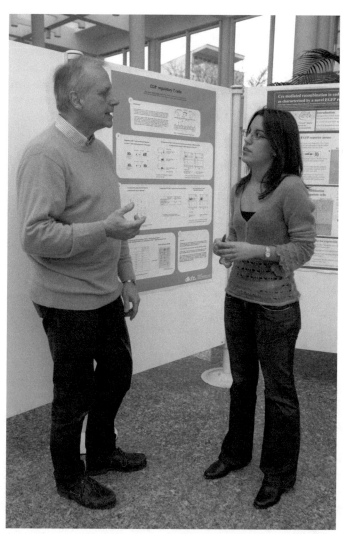

Maria is impressed with the supervision by her group leader, Prof. Bernd Arnold

are financed directly by the divisions from their own external resources. When seeking suitable candidates, they are often all too pleased to consider candidates from the pool of the PhD program, who, after all, have already successfully passed one selection round.

Incidentally, the further-education courses provided within the PhD program have, since October 2004, also become compulsory for externally funded doctoral students, since the Heidelberg faculties now make the award of a doctoral degree dependent on having attended such courses.

Maria Papatriantafyllou decided, after talking to Professor Bernd Arnold, to begin her

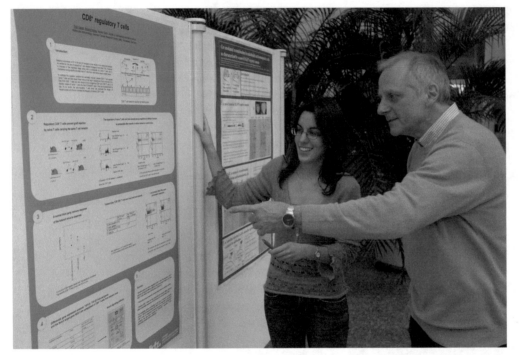

Furthermore the privileged divisional heads have a price to pay: "Each of those who acquired a doctoral student in the previous round has to take part in the next selection process as an assessor", explains Thomas Efferth.

Intensive Supervision Guaranteed

A few months after her successful interview, Maria moved to Heidelberg. She was happy to find that the moderately sized town on the Neckar – in contrast to her native Athens – no longer entailed a one-and-a-half-hour each-way journey to work. Her start was made easy by helpful colleagues and because she had already been learning German for three years. She is especially enthusiastic about the support she received from her group leader Bernd Arnold. To make sure that no problems arise in this respect, the PhD program has strict rules: For every student

doctoral work in his research group within the Division of Molecular Immunology. In order to set the wheels in motion, her future supervisor had to submit the plans for her doctoral research project to the staff committee. The Scientific Council of the Center decides about the applications.

Doctoral positions within the PhD program are highly sought after in the Center, since they require no funding from the divisional budget. To avoid internal wrangling about the distribution of these positions, there is a rule that each year the program allocates no more than one position per division.

there is a responsible 'advisory committee' comprising three persons, the personal supervisor and two other scientists, of whom at least one must be from a different division. Each year the students submit a report on their work to their supervisor. This is intended to demonstrate whether the research project is progressing successfully and whether it can be completed within a reasonable time. Sponsorship by the PhD program is limited to a period of three years.

"The PhD program brings benefits for both sides", says Thomas Efferth. "The students can be sure that they are gaining a first-class scientific training and excellent supervision of their work. The DKFZ, in turn, attracts outstanding applicants from throughout the world." Efferth is a proven expert on academic educational projects. Before becoming head of the International PhD Program, he coordinated the advanced study course 'Molecular Cell Biology' of the University of Heidelberg, and prior to that he was managing director of the Virtual University Rhineland-Palatinate. Currently he is working to increase international awareness of the DKFZ program so that – unlike Maria Papatriantafyllou – students don't have to rely on a lucky mouse click in order to find out about the opportunities offered by the Center. Efferth is sending leaflets and posters to about 1000 universities around the world and has placed announcements in the journal *Science*.

What about German students? With so much international competition, do they have any chance at all of gaining a place on the PhD program? "Yes, definitely", emphasizes Efferth. "Only about 30 percent of our applicants are Germans, but they account for roughly 50 percent of the participants. The German students are simply very good."

Sibylle Kohlstädt

Learning by Doing – At the Heidelberg Life Science Lab High School Students Design Their Own Experiments

High flyers such as Philipp Börsch-Supan are no exception at the Heidelberg Life Science Lab: He began his scientific career in the 9th grade with a school chemistry project. The topic: Compostable plastics. One year later, while Philipp was living with his parents in New England, USA, he encountered lobsters, or, more precisely, their shells. This material, considered exotic in this part of the world, is such a common waste product in New England that it presents disposal problems. Philipp soon had the idea of testing the shell of these articulated animals as a possible starting material for biodegradable plastics. A short time afterwards, this work earned him first place in the Rhineland-Palatinate section of the youth research competition 'Jugend forscht', and a

fourth place in the national competition.

In 2004, after completing the 12th grade, Philipp applied to the Heidelberg Life Science Lab. Dr. Thomas Schutz, the initiator and head of the Lab, had, from the very beginning, the student with the proven expertise in chemistry in mind for a special project. Many of the Lab participants would like to independently pursue scientific questions, but are lacking the requisite theoretical and practical know-how. Philipp's task should be to help them as advisor. His crustacean project had led him to ask new questions: Why do lobsters turn red when they are cooked? More accurately, what causes the pigment crustacyanin, originally blue, to change its color when heated? Philipp was able to organize a working place in the learning laboratory of the Heidelberg EXPLO. Centered on the analysis of the lobster pigments he devised a practical course that was open to all Lab participants who

wanted to learn about biochemical techniques. He also included instruction concerning how to search the scientific literature, where to find the 'recipes' for biochemical analysis, and how to construct scientific hypotheses.

Learning Through Teaching

Philipp's activities at the Life Science Lab have already been successful on two accounts: A Lab participant is now independently analyzing blood proteins from stick insects. And Philipp, who long ago moved on to address new problems, is entering the competition 'Jugend forscht' for a second time, this time with the results of an analysis of jelly-fish pigments – a project in which he is being supported by protein analysts from the German Cancer Research Center. "Philipp's project combines the central pedagogical demands that we have set ourselves with the Life Science Lab", explains Thomas Schutz.

In the physics working group of the Heidelberg Life Science Lab, high school students independently study the theoretical foundations of their experiments

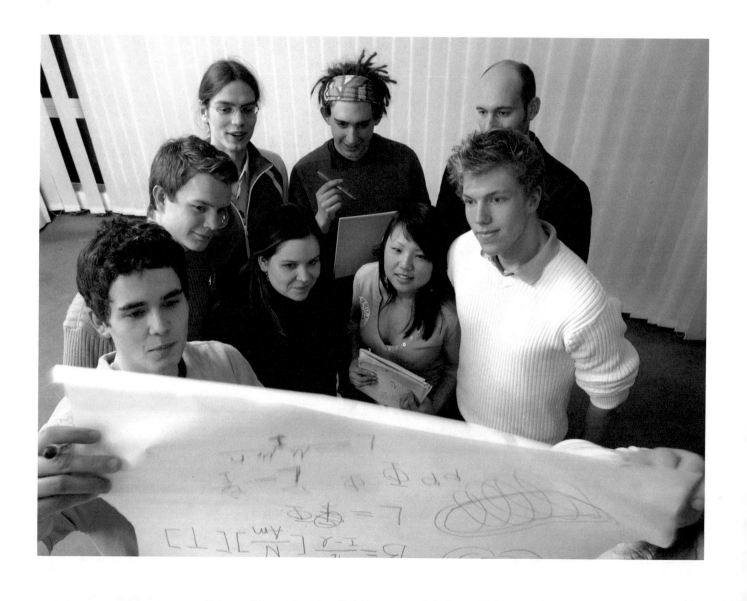

"The participants gain not only specialist skills and fundamental knowledge, but also learn the relevant methodology. They work on a real research project and not on an invented problem, as is mostly the case in school science lessons. In addition they acquire further knowledge and skills through teaching others, e.g. in the presentation of their results to the working group. Here, as a matter of course, they adopt the appropriate technical forms of presentation and discourse."

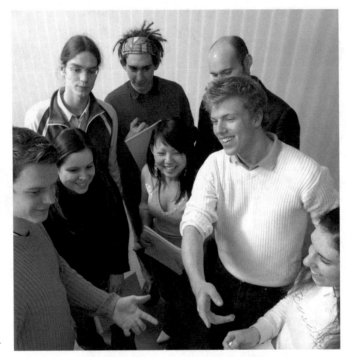

The Heidelberg Life Science Lab (LSL) has existed since 1999. Today it is financed for the most part by its supporting organization, the Deutsches Krebsforschungszentrum. In addition, it applies for and receives its own external funding as well as sponsorship funds. From the 8th grade upwards, school students interested in natural sciences can apply to the Lab by holding a short talk. Those chosen to participate – at present 188 students – are entitled to take part in all the various activities of the LSL. Philipp Börsch-Supan's lobster practical is to be found in the category 'inter-working-group project' and is among the most highly evolved of the activities offered by the lab. In parallel with these activities, there is a whole range of other events. The basis is formed by the Friday lectures at the Center, which surprise their audiences with a broad spectrum of topics: From 'Stem cells and cancer' and 'Ornithological prospects for the Wadden Sea ecosystem' the lectures extend to

Helge Baumann (right) is one of the two student mentors of the physics working group

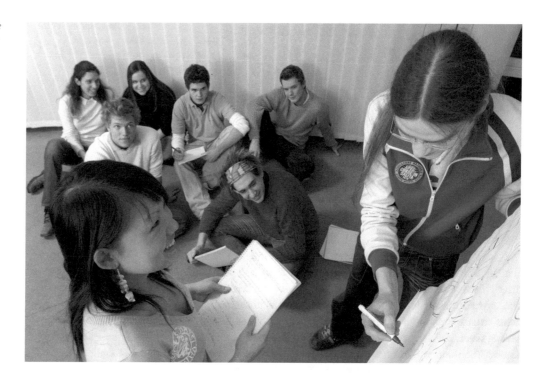

topics such as 'Tactile sensors in robotics' or a 'Philosophical approach to the concept of naturalness in medicine'. These events are open to the general public and are especially popular with teachers.

The participants of the Life Science Labs, who meet regularly on Friday afternoons for the lectures, mostly live in Baden-Württemberg or the neighboring states Hesse and Rhineland-Palatinate. But a few even make the long journey from

Saxony and North Rhine-Westphalia. "Attendance is not compulsory, but the Friday sessions give an important rhythm to the LSL: The students arrange their other Lab activities around this regular meeting", explains Thomas Schultz.

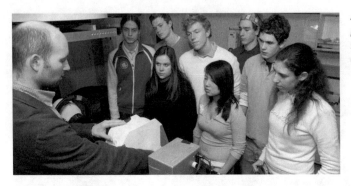

Andreas Rau, scientific mentor of the physics working group, with his students during a visit at the linear accelerator

Seminars, Science Academies, and Working Groups

The Life Science Lab also organizes weekend seminars and, during the summer holidays, holds science academies lasting several weeks, in Germany or abroad. The main work of the LSL, however, is invested in the working groups (WGs). In these the Life Science Lab cooperates, among others, with the universities of Heidelberg and Mannheim, or with the European Molecular Biology Laboratory. The scientific institutes, including of course the German Cancer Research Center as supporting organization, provide the infrastructure within which the students themselves organize their regular and independent project work. Every Lab participant has to join one scientific WG; the choice at present is among biochemistry, chemistry, computer science, mathematics, molecular biology, neuropsychology, pharmacy, physics, and zoology. In addition there is a philosophy WG, whose topics such as ethics, epistemology, and anthropology are linked to scientific problems.

The coordination point for the physics WG is the DKFZ. The project was initiated by Professor Wolfgang Schlegel, head of the division "Medical Physics in Radiology". The task: to test a new tracking system, designed to follow the position of a tumor during involuntary movement, due for example to breathing or intestinal motor activity. This 'Online Tumor Tracking System' which continually transmits the position of the tumor to special measuring antennas, was developed by an American company and is just now being approved for medical use. The role of scientific mentor for the physics WG has been taken on by Andreas Rau. As part of his doctoral studies at the DKFZ he will investigate

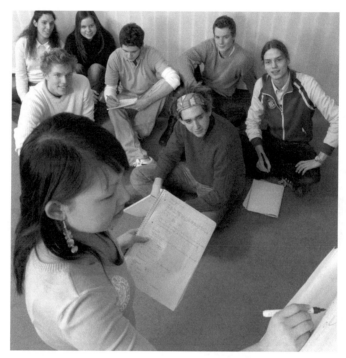

WGs have a coordinating function: they fix the dates for group activities and make relevant scientific information available to the group on the Lab's own internet platform. A student mentor is also responsible for the presentation of the WG's results within the Life Science Lab and also suggests a direction for the project work. Each WG receives further guidance from teacher mentors.

'Real' Research in the WGs

"The physics WG is impatiently waiting for the tracking system to arrive so that they can start the practical tests at last", says Helge. By that time the students are well prepared for their task. On their own they took steps to acquire the necessary background knowledge: What kind of radiation is used in cancer treatment? What effect precisely does it have on cancer cells? How can one guide the radiation exactly onto the tracking? How is

whether this tracking system is suited for use in radiotherapy. One of the two student mentors of the WG is Helge Baumann, in the 13th grade, who has been a member of the Life Science Lab for four years. He has been involved in the tumor tracking project from the outset. The student mentors of the

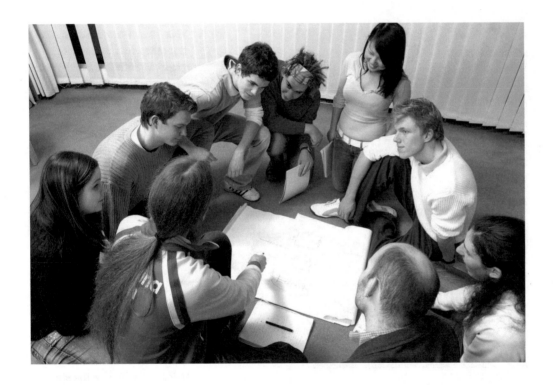

radiotherapy planned in three dimensions? Together with their scientific mentor, the students visited the linear accelerator and the radiological diagnostic equipment. At the Bunsen Gymnasium, a neighboring school, they were able to perform experiments that help to demonstrate the physical foundations for their planned series of measurements. As soon as the tracking system arrives at the DKFZ, the WG can begin their measurements. The plan is that the students should investigate how the measuring accuracy of the system is influenced by magnetic field perturbations caused by the linear accelerator. Asked whether he would rely on the results gathered by the students, Andreas Rau replies: "For sure that is my intention. They are so well prepared, and of course the whole idea is that they should work independently." A member of the WG explains why his group is so committed to the project: "What we are doing here is not just anything; we are involved in forefront problems of medical physics. Tumor tracking is *the* hot topic in radiotherapy. To be part of this work is far more motivating than being a spectator at some demonstration experiment."

Find out more about the Heidelberg Life Science Lab: http://life-science-lab.xmachina.de/

Sybille Kohlstädt

The Magic Formula for Inducing Tobacco Addiction

"Nicotine plus high pH value. That's the magic formula." Dr. Martina Pötschke-Langer has a simple answer to the question why cigarettes are addictive. "And the trick with the pH value has made the road to addiction even shorter."

Nicotine is the principal addictive substance in tobacco. Manufacturers realized were soon that it is primarily the addictive potential of this neurotoxic substance that keeps smokers smoking despite the sure perspective of the most severe diseases. Therefore, the tobacco industry has a natural interest in a high bioavailability of nicotine in their products. "For the manufacturers, a cigarette is nothing but a kind of nicotine delivery device", criticizes Pötschke-Langer, a doctor who leads the Division of Cancer Prevention at the DKFZ. And

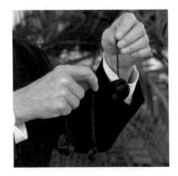

pH manipulation allows them to increase the doses delivered at will. The higher – i.e. the more basic – the pH value of tobacco smoke, the more nicotine is present in its free form, not bound to salts in a molecule complex. Only free nicotine is rapidly absorbed by the body to give the smoker the desired "kick", i.e. the rapid rise of the levels of this pharmacologically highly active toxic. This pH dependence was used by ingenious chemists of the tobacco industry to specifically increase the bioavailability of nicotine by manipulating the acid-base equilibrium. One way is to add ammonia components

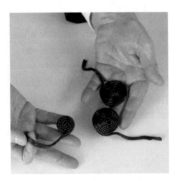

to the tobacco; another, simpler and "natural" way, so to speak, is through nitrate fertilization of the tobacco plants.

The most wonderful thing for cigarette makers: This manipulation does not increase the total nicotine content that is printed on every cigarette package. Thus, the public, who has been concerned about the health hazards of smoking ever since the 1950s despite all reassuring statements by the tobacco industry, has been deliberately deceived with seemingly low nicotine yields.

Licorice, cocoa, peppermint: Who would expect these sweets in tobacco smoke? Dr. Martina Pötschke-Langer and Prof. Heinz Walter Thielmann are screening US tobacco industry documents for information pointing to such additives

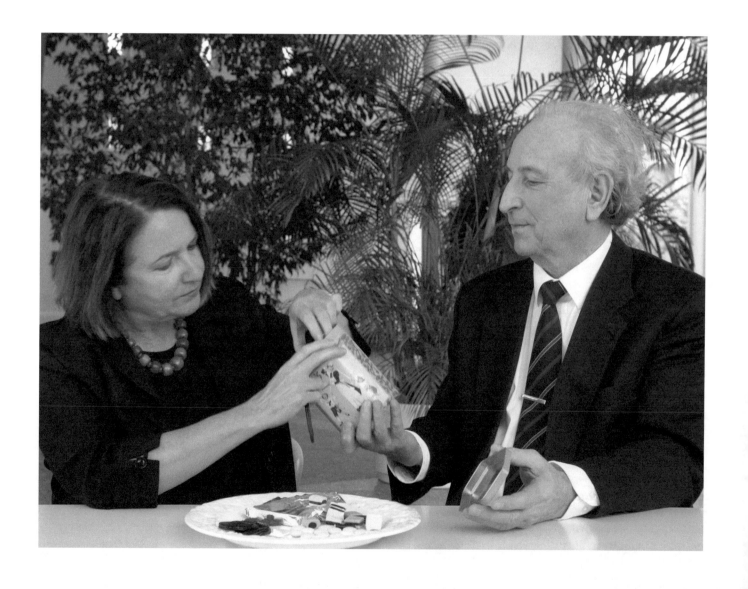

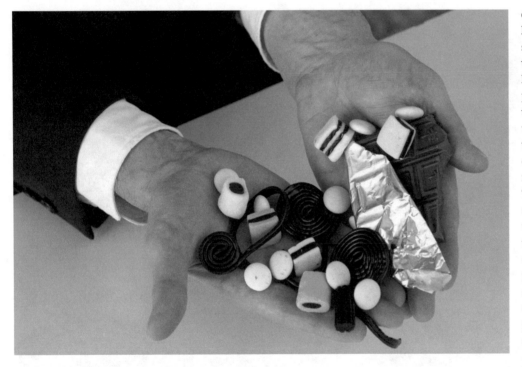

documents. The scientists were looking for written evidence showing how tobacco manufacturers had deliberately manipulated the qualities of their products by using additives. Up to 600 different additives are used; they can constitute up to ten percent of the total weight of the cigarette. During their research, Pötschke-Langer and Thielmann soon discovered the strategy behind tobacco product manipulation: Increasing the addiction and making it easier to inhale the smoke, in particular, in order to make smoking easier for beginning smokers. Thus, the cigarette product became even more dangerous than it already was.

Ammonia to Enhance Addictiveness

The Marlboro brand is a success story of this strategy: Phillip Morris was able to triple sales of the "Cowboy brand" between 1960 and 1975, which the tobacco industry itself attributes to the threefold increase of the ratio of free nicotine contained in the cigarette over the same period of time. "The secret of Marlboro is ammonia." This statement is found in the tobacco industry documents that had to be made publicly available according to a 1998 settlement between the US Attorney General and the US tobacco companies.

Jointly with biochemist Professor Heinz Walter Thielmann, staff members of Pötschke-Langer's division have systematically searched through these

Menthol cigarettes, the ones with the "cool" flavor, have been on the market since the 1950s. But almost all "regular" cigarettes also contain the substance at levels between 0.01 and 0.03 percent of weight. This is below the threshold at which a smoker consciously perceives the chemical with the typical peppermint flavor. Menthol is added to tobacco chiefly because of its pain relieving qualities. In the mouth and throat it acts like a local anesthetic that makes inhaling the smoke less irritating. Thus, deeper inhalation into the lungs becomes possible and the smoke reaches the deep bronchial branches of the lung. In internal industry documents, cigarette makers sometimes refer to menthol as a "smoke soother". In addition, menthol stimulates the cold receptors in the mouth mucosa, thus causing a sense of freshness that covers the irritation by the harsh tobacco smoke. Moreover, a sensory stimulus caused by menthol inhalation leads to an increased breathing frequency and volume so that more smoke is inhaled more rapidly and deeper.

Permitted Poisons

Surprisingly, these manipulations are not legally prohibited – quite the opposite: The Tobacco Product Regulation of the German Food and Commodities Act (Lebensmittel- und Bedarfsgegenständegesetz, LMBG) contains a detailed list of what manufacturers are allowed to add to tobacco. Alongside a list of substances which reads like the contents list of a chemistry experimentation set, there is a host of harmless sounding substances that one would expect as ingredients of confectionery,

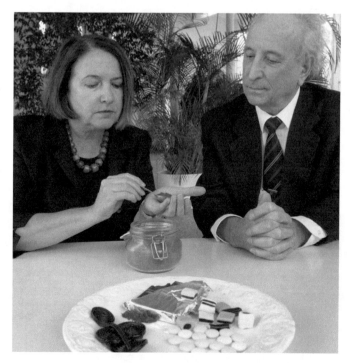

but not as additives to tobacco products: Maple syrup, licorice, cocoa, vanilla or molasses are used to give an enjoyable, sweet flavor to the smoke. "This is a fundamental mistake of the Tobacco Regulation", says Heinz Walter Thielmann. "The legislator assumes that since these substances are approved for use in food, they cannot be harmful in tobacco products. A totally absurd assumption, for the chemistry at temperatures on the kitchen stove is not comparable to what is going on at 600 to 900 degrees in the glowing cone of a cigarette." At such heat, most of the additives are converted into a multitude of pyrolysis products. These pyrolysis products determine the toxic potential of the inhaled smoke, while the additives in their original form are usually responsible only for a minor part of toxicity. Thus, among the permitted tobacco additives, there are a lot of precursors of carcinogenic substances to be found. Thielmann explains: "Another

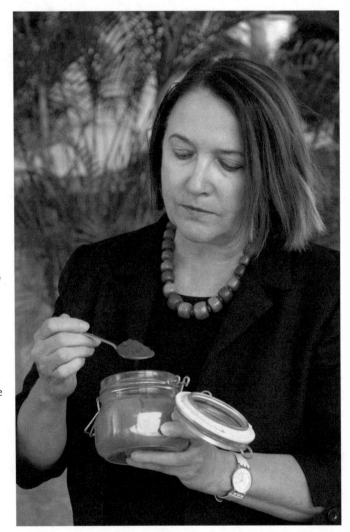

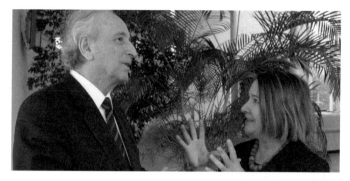

problem is that chemically undefined mixtures such as fruit juice, honey or wood give manufacturers almost infinite freedom in designing their products." Burning of many of these permitted additives increases the content of carcinogenic polycyclic hydrocarbons. Manipulation of the pH value also makes the cigarette even more carcinogenic. The high nitrate content of tobacco plants or added ammonia compounds increase the proportion of carcinogenic N-nitrosamines and aromatic amines. Some of the explicitly permitted tobacco additives have been classified as directly carcinogenic, even without pyrolysis. Examples include glyoxal, azo dyes and salts of cobalt.

Smooth Smoke Makes It Easier to Start Smoking

"The most terrible thing is", says Martina Pötschke-Langer, "that the deliberate product manipulations have turned the cigarette market into a children's market." The average age of the beginning smoker continues to drop and is presently at 13 to 14 years. Eleven percent of juvenile smokers have smoked their first cigarette before they turned 11 years. No wonder, with menthol soothing the pain and all kinds of sweet stuff making the harsh smoke tolerable. "The beginning smoker and inhaler has a low tolerance for smoke irritation, hence the smoke should be as bland as possible", it reads in a 1974 RJ Reynolds document. Consequently, the tobacco giant adjusted the product qualities of its best-selling "Camel" brand to the model of Marlboro, which was the most popular youth brand well into the 1970s.

Germany, alongside Belgium and the UK, is among the few countries in the EU which have clearly regulated the ingredients for cigarettes in a tobacco regulation. Therefore, Martina Pötschke-Langer fears that the German regulation might be taken over Europe-wide without further examination. "But we have to achieve the exact opposite: All ingredients that contribute to addictiveness and make smoking easier need to be prohibited promptly." The Federal Ministry of Food, Agriculture and Consumer Protection has decided in Spring 2005 that all additives will be examined to determine their hazardous potential. For Pötschke-Langer, this is by far not enough: "A whole number of additives have long since been assessed, for example by the MAK Commission or the International Agency for Research on Cancer (IARC) in Lyon. For these, the legislator could take immediate action by prohibiting them without delay."

Sibylle Kohlstädt

The Wish to Have Children in Spite of Cancer

"Well, and in December, I will become a father." Normally, this piece of news would encourage spontaneous congratulations. If it comes from a cancer patient whose disease – a chronic form of myeloic leukemia (CML) – has been considered to date as hard to control, then even experienced staff of the telephone cancer information service KID hesitate.

This also happened to the KID staff member who received this call by an expectant father. In view of the so far relatively poor prognosis of CML patients, the topic of children and pregnancy had only rarely been raised.

However, this patient had been receiving a new drug for some time. US molecular biologist Brian J. Druker and his collegues succeeded in specifically interfering with the defective cellular processes in chronic myeloic leukemia. Imatinib, the drug with the trade name Glivec that was developed on the basis of his research, appears to really slow down the disease in the long term and was approved in Europe in late 2001.

Research Changes Quality of Life

Although the caller had mentioned the topic of offspring only in passing, the KID staff member requested information from the KID research team about Glivec and the wish to have children. The research team at KID is not only responsible for feeding the internal knowledge database – the basis for answering questions – with up-to-date, scientifically well founded information. In the case of new developments or very specific questions, the staff of the research team will also directly search for literature sources, contacts, or addresses.

Several years prior to this call, when first clinical trials of Imatinib had been successful and media reports – even articles about the manufacturer's stock exchange quotation – lead to enquiries at the cancer information service, KID had entered a text about the substance into the database and updated it when the drug received approval.

Search for Information Worldwide

However, the search for scientific literature on the topic of pregnancy and Glivec provided no results. It was in patients' forums and chats that KID finally found some information: Here, many sufferers from the US, Canada and also from Germany had exchanged information about how the new drug opened up new prospects for them. They felt so good that even long-term life and family planning seemed to be possible once more. Shortly afterwards,

New drugs open up new prospects for life and family planning for cancer patients. Encouraged by questions from callers, KID explored the data situation concerning the topic "The wish to have a child despite cancer"

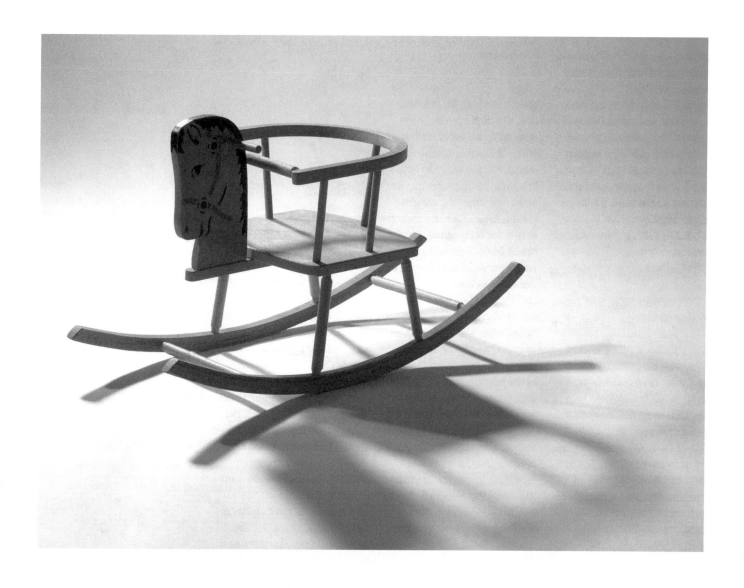

KID staff learned in their information service of first patients who had ventured pregnancy while receiving Glivec – despite explicit warnings in the package insert and much to the dismay of the manufacturer, who only learned about this from KID staff members. It was not until 2005 that specialist publications on the topic finally became available; these were included in KID's information collection.

Taking up Ideas

The substance Glivec is only one example of how advances in cancer research change not only "hard" parameters such as survival time, but also less tangible ones such as quality of life of those affected. Thus, the wish to have children is a topic that has come up in recent years in the calls or e-mails of patients with other tumor types, too. In Winter 2003, KID posted a comprehensive information text on this topic on its Internet site.

When searching for information, KID research staff have been using a host of contacts, which the cancer information service has been able to establish since its inception two decades ago. Thus, the competence networks for leukemia research, for lymphomas and for cancer in children and young adults provided valuable ideas. The German breast cancer study group, German Breast Group, also came forward with information about topics such as cancer diagnosis during pregnancy. Experts on the topic of the wish to have children after cancer from the disciplines of gynecology and oncology as well as experts in the follow-up care of childhood cancer survivors offered further education events for the team. KID reciprocated with a short qualitative evelution of the spectrum of enquiries on this topic on the basis of its anon-

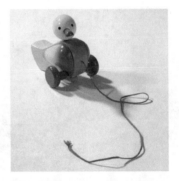

ymous documentation of incoming calls and e-mails.

Feedback for the Specialists

Even for specialists, an evaluation of several hundred thousand contacts provides unusually deep insights into the questions and problems of cancer patients. The enquiries are often about topics which the patients are reluctant to mention in conversation with their doctors; they often concern matters that become relevant after treatment is concluded and contact to the hospital or doctor's office becomes more sporadic. Many enquiries also reflect how confusing the structures of the health service sometimes are for laypersons. Therefore, KID has effectively taken on a guiding role, providing information, based on more than 3,000 cancer-related addresses in its database, on where to find relevant contacts for the individual questions.

Not Only Patients Are a Target Group for Information

Approximately one half of the enquiries at KID come from persons who are often left out of the general education about the topic of cancer and for whom the simple advice, "Ask your doctor", is not useful: family and friends. It is them who often have an enormous need for information, because they wish to support the patient as best they can, but are usually excluded from contact to expert care givers. Their calls and e-mails show that they, too, tend to need psychological support in this difficult period of their

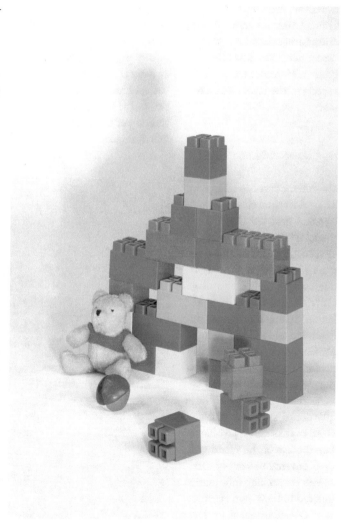

lives. And: More often than the average, they are interested in cancer prevention and early cancer detection. KID offers profound information on these aspects of the topic of cancer, too.

High User Satisfaction

The Internet service offered by KID – www.krebsinforma-tion.de – does not substitute the telephone information service. Instead, it is intended to enable users to pose the right questions to their doctor or other experts. However, in a survey among KID callers conducted in 2005, the wish for a personal conversation with a doctor or a telephone information service was expressed by more than 80 percent of those questioned and, thus, still clearly ranks first – just like before the age of the World Wide Web. Seventy percent of KID callers are seeking information tailored to their own specific case. Questions about general

information and classification are significantly less frequent. By far the most important quality expected from KID by 83 percent of users is a good subject knowledge. To ensure this in the long term, further training of the staff is undertaken at regular intervals to up-

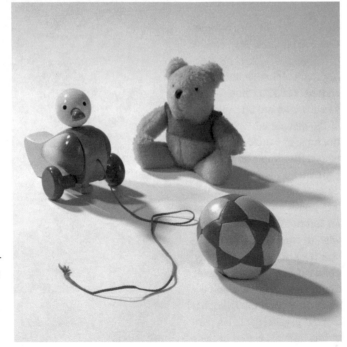

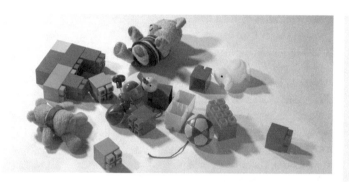

date their knowledge. However, the empathy which KID staff use in their conversations with persons seeking information by telephone, e-mail or in the consulting service can hardly be learned by training: Anybody who wants to work for KID – just needs to have it.

Birgit Hiller

The cancer information service KID was launched in 1986 at the German Cancer Research Center. The service, which provides information for the public nationwide, is funded by the German Ministry of Health; the State of Baden-Wuerttemberg also contributes to the funding.

Cancer Information Service:
Monday through Friday,
8 am to 8 pm,
phone ++49 (0) 6221 41 0121

Breast Cancer Hotline:
Monday through Friday,
8 am to 8 pm,
phone ++49 (0) 6221 42 4343

Cancer Pain Information Service:
Monday through Friday,
noon to 4 pm,
phone ++49 (0) 6221 42 2000

Fatigue Hotline:
Monday, Wednesday, Friday,
4 pm to 7 pm, phone ++49
(0) 6221 42 4344

E-Mail-Service:
krebsinformation@dkfz.de

KID on the Internet:
www.krebsinformation.de,
cancer pain: www.ksid.de

Appointments for the KID consulting service offered at the National Center for Tumor Diseases (NCT) can be scheduled at ++49 (0) 6221 56 4801 or at tagesklinik_nct@med.uni-heidelberg.de

Heidelberg as the Hub of a Worldwide Cancer Research Network

The trend towards globalization has continued unabated in recent years. In the meantime the term has become a fashionable buzzword in many domains of life. In science, however, the upkeep of international relationships is far more than just a fashion. The German Cancer Research Center would be hard to imagine without its personal and scientific exchange with researchers at home and abroad, who have themselves spent lengthy periods at the Center. Professor Peter Bannasch began in 2002 to develop an alumni program at the DKFZ. It aims to give the Center's former researchers the opportunity, after completing their research stay, to remain informed about current activities and to follow the progress of the research work they began in Heidelberg.

The seed of this Alumni Program has existed for a long time: Many scientists from the Center have for years maintained contact to former colleagues from around the world, joining forces with them to form international teams. At present the Center is the place of work for approximately 200 foreign scientists, whose stays are financed by a variety of fellowship programs, for example, the guest scientist program or the international PhD program of the DKFZ, the Humboldt Foundation, or the German Academic Exchange Service, or from project funds.

It is almost a tradition that the staff of the DKFZ accompany the guest scientist on excursions to explore the Rhine-Neckar region and learn about its people, places, and cultural attractions – for example, visiting the BASF plant in Ludwigshafen, or undertaking a historical tour of the town Speyer. In addition, regular scientific meetings, held both at the Center and in the home countries of the guests, provide the chance to meet again in person.

A special highlight was the first general alumni meeting held at the beginning of June 2004. It attracted 150 participants including researchers from China, USA and Europe, who met to present their research results and to learn about the main current research activities at the Center. On the first day some of the former DKFZ staff presented their latest results on the pathobiology of cancer cells and on the role of immunological processes in defending the body against cancer. The second day was given over to scientists from the Center, who reported on the results of their own research. This meeting was occasion for the decision to found the DKFZ Alumni Association (Alumni Deutsches Krebsforschungszentrum Heidelberg e.V.) – a further building block for the alumni program. A top priority for the as-

Time for conversation in a relaxed atmosphere: Heike Langlotz with two alumni, Dr. Ilia Toshkov and Dr. Yun Niu

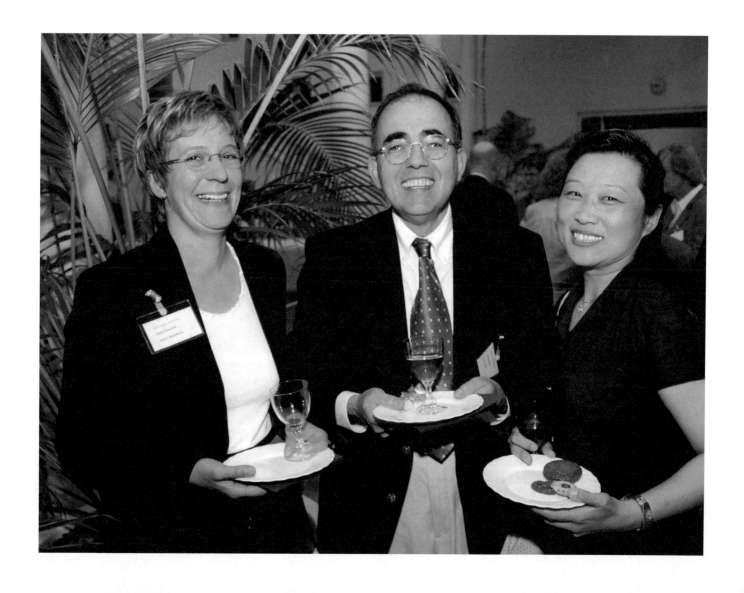

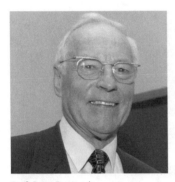

Prof. Peter Bannasch

sociation is to support young scientists by facilitating research visits and helping to establish collaborations. From the start, the pathologist Peter Bannasch has been the driving force behind the alumni program and also worked to prepare the ground for this fragile young enterprise. In the meantime he has been elected as chairman of the newly founded association. He is supported by Scientific Director Professor Otmar D. Wiestler, Dr. Konrad Buschbeck, a retired ministerial advisor and longstanding former member of the DKFZ Board of Trustees, and Elfriede Mang, the secretary of the association.

Twice yearly the association issues a newsletter, which is specially designed to provide information of interest to alumni. The first issue of 'Alumni Deutsches Krebsforschungszentrum' appeared in English in the fall of 2003. The newsletter, which reports on current progress in research at the DKFZ and on developments in international relations, helps to maintain long-term contacts to former visiting scientists, scientists, and doctoral students of the Center.

A topic focused on in the first issue was the 'Sino-German Workshop on Cancer and Infectious Diseases' in Beijing, which was jointly organized with the German Research Center for Biotechnology (GBF), Brunswick. The co-organizer on the Chinese side was the Chinese Academy of Medical Sciences (CAMS). This event provided the framework for the signing of a memorandum concerning the future cooperation between the Helmholtz Asso-

ciation and CAMS. Representatives of the Cancer Research Center and the GBF reported on their latest research results in various rounds of presentations. A visit to the research laboratories at the CAMS cancer clinic together with final round-table discussions gave the DKFZ delegation the opportunity to forge some initial scientific contacts. These contacts have already borne fruit, such as the start of several small joint projects. Furthermore, at the institutional level there are plans to establish a program of collaboration between the German Cancer Research Center and the Chinese Cancer Institute, in particular in relation to the support of young scientists through exchange programs.

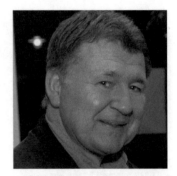

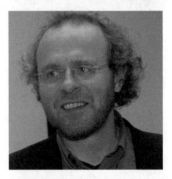

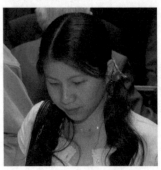

Right, from top: Prof. Mihály Bak,
Prof. Thomas Boehm, Dr. Ying Ying

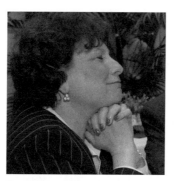

Ilana Lowi

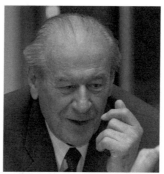

Prof. Mieczyslaw Chorazy

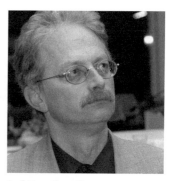

Prof. Hans-Georg Rammensee

Before the workshop took place, the first meeting of the DKFZ Alumni Association was held under the leadership of Peter Bannasch. Among other things, it provided an opportunity to meet and converse personally with Chinese applicants for the International PhD-program of the DKFZ. In addition, a Chinese DKFZ Alumni Club was founded, and Professor Qin Su (CAMS) was elected as its coordinator. In between the large meetings in Heidelberg, other smaller events are planned abroad. DKFZ receptions as fringe events at major scientific meetings and congresses offer the Alumni an ideal opportunity not only to renew their friendships and scientific contacts to former colleagues, but also to become acquainted with new colleagues.

The sum of these activities should lead to the creation of a world-wide network that promotes and stimulates national and international cooperations in cancer research. However, openness in all directions as well as active support are needed to ensure that the seed germinates and grows into a flourishing enterprise.

Dagmar Anders

Award-Winning Research

2006

Dr. Ana Martin-Villalba, Division of Immunogenetics, was awarded the newly established **Paul Ehrlich and Ludwig Darmstaedter Young Scientists' Award** in March 2006. The scientist showed that blocking CD95-mediated apoptosis in mice can reduce the effects of surgically induced paralysis. Four weeks after such treatment, mice were able to move their legs again, while untreated animals remained paralyzed. Earlier, Martin-Villalba

had shown that blocking CD95-mediated apoptosis after a stroke can help save cells and prevent consequences such as paralyses. The award is worth 60 000 euros.

2005

Professor Harald zur Hausen, former Chairman of the Management Board and Scientific Director of the Center, was awarded the **Prince Mahidol Award** in December 2005. Zur Hausen receives the prize, worth 50 000 US dollars, for his contributions to public health care. Furthermore, zur Hausen received the **13th Raymond Bour-**

gine Award in February 2006 and was honored with the Medal of Merit of the State of Baden-Wuerttemberg in April 2006. Since the 1970s, zur Hausen focused his research mainly on papillomaviruses. He was the first to discover that individual types of these viruses, which were first isolated in his working group, can cause cervical cancer. This discovery paved the way for novel prevention measures. Thus, a vaccine against papillomaviruses is available since Summer 2006.

Professor Heike Allgayer, head of the Clinical Cooperation Unit "Molecular Oncology of Solid Tumors", was awarded the 2005 **Alfried Krupp Award** for young university lecturers. Allgayer, a surgeon and molecular biologist, has been studying the mechanisms that turn tumor cells into invasive metastases. She discovered a central role of the urokinase receptor (uPAR): Tumor cells which form this molecule on their surface are able to colonize other tis-

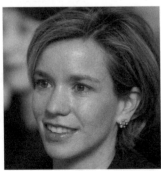
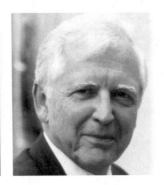
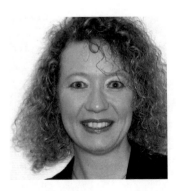

sues. Expression of the receptor also facilitates predictions about the further course of the disease. Heike Allgayer also investigated the genetic regulation of uPAR and discovered that the activation pathways for the production of the protein in cancer cells differ from those in normal cells. Thus, gene regulation is another level at which it is possible to determine whether tumor cells have the potential to metastasize.

The Krupp Award is worth one million euros. The prize money is issued to the winner over a period of five years.

Professor Christof von Kalle, director of the National Center for Tumor Diseases (NCT) Heidelberg and head of the Division of Translational Oncology at the DKFZ, was awarded, jointly with three colleagues, the 2005 **Langen Science Award** worth 10 000 euros. The scientists were able to increase the safety of gene therapy for treating severe combined immunodeficiency disease (SCID), a life-threatening hereditary disease. Several of the treated children had developed leukemia after gene therapy. Von Kalle and colleagues have developed a method for determining the site where the thera-

peutic gene has inserted itself into the genetic material. Thus, it is possible to check whether oncogenes may be activated as a result of the gene insertion.

Dr. Amir Abdollahi (foto bottom) of the Clinical Cooperation Unit "Radiation Oncology" was the recipient of the 2005 **Walther and Christine Richtzenhain Dissertation Prize**. He studied the cellular signaling pathways by which endostatin regulates the formation of new blood vessels. Abdollahi shares the prize with **Dr. Dr. Christian Thieke**, who, during his PhD research at the Division of Medical Physics in Radiation Oncol-

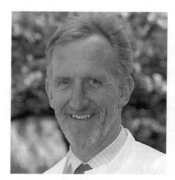
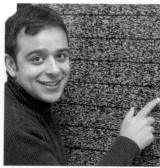

ogy, has developed methods to improve computer assisted planning in precision radiotherapy.

2004

Dr. Angela Risch, Division of Toxicology and Cancer Risk Factors, was awarded the **Dr. Emil Salzer Award** in 2004. Risch, a biochemist, received the EUR 5,000 cash prize for her investigation of genetic variants of the cytochrome P450 enzymes which mediate an increased lung cancer risk.

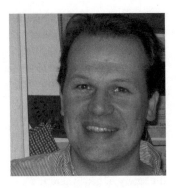

The newly established **Sibylle Assmus Prize** was awarded jointly to **Dr. Bernhard Radlwimmer** (foto top), Division of Molecular Genetics, and Dr. Christel Herold-Mende of the University Neurosurgical Hospital in Heidelberg. The two scientists identified clinically relevant markers in stem cell populations of malignant brain tumors.

Dr. Markus Feuerer and **Dr. Philipp Beckhove** of the Division of Cellular Immunology discovered that the bone marrow is a location of a primary T cell response to cancer cells. For this discovery, they received the 2004 **Walther and Christine Richtzenhain Prize**, a cash award worth 10 000 euros.

Jointly with their colleague, PD **Dr. Viktor Umansky**, the two researchers had also received the **Sir Hans Krebs Prize** for the advancement of basic medical research back in 2002. The prize is worth 20 000 euros.

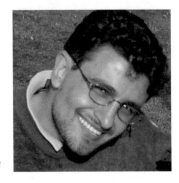

Hassan Adwan of the Research Group "Toxicology and Chemotherapy" was awarded the **Bondronat Prize** Class I for young scientists under age 35, which consists of a cash gift of 10 000 euros. Adwan demonstrated that growth and migration of breast cancer cells can be influenced using antisense oligonucleotides against the genes of bone sialoprotein and osteopontin. Thus, he discovered a novel approach for treating breast cancer metastases. The prize is awarded by the company Hoffmann-LaRoche for contributions to the improvement of breast cancer treatment.

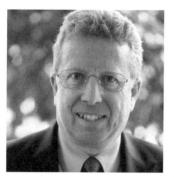

Professor Dietrich Keppler, head of the Division of Tumor Biochemistry, was honored for his life's work with the 2003 **Lucie Bolte Award**. The Lucie Bolte Foundation presents this award to honor important achievements in the area of liver research. Dietrich Keppler focused his scientific career on investigating the pathogenesis and pathochemistry of liver diseases. In recent years, he elucidated the molecular transport processes of liver cells.

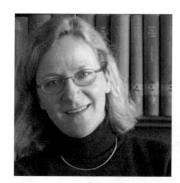

Jointly with colleagues from the University of Saarland, **Dr. Clarissa Gerhäuser**, Division of Toxicology and Cancer Risk Factors, and her working group received the 2003 **Phoenix Pharma Science Award** worth 5,000 euros. The scientists were honored for the discovery of xanthohumol, a substance obtained from hop, which has shown a cancer-preventive effect in cellular test systems. Pharmaceutical wholesaler Phoenix Pharmahandel awards this prize for outstanding

achievements in pharmacological and pharmaceutical research.

The winner of the 2003 **German Cancer Aid Award** was **Professor Peter Lichter**, head of the Division of Molecular Genetics. The prize, worth 10 000 euros, is awarded by the German Cancer Aid (Deutsche Krebshilfe) on behalf of the Dr. Wilhelm Hoffmann family to honor researchers whose work contributes to the fight against cancer. In 2002, Peter Lichter had already received the experimental part of the **German Cancer Award**, which the Deutsche Krebsgesellschaft

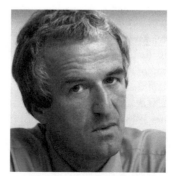

awarded to honor his internationally acclaimed work relating to fast and comprehensive genome analysis. Fluorescence in situ hybridization (FISH) and matrix-based comparative genomic hybridization (matrix CGH) are two analysis methods developed by Lichter that are commonly used in cancer research today. FISH closed a gap between cytological research and genomics. Using fluorescent dyes, the technology has made it possible to visualize any section of the genome directly in the tumor tissue. Matrix CGH involves the simultaneous use of genomes of tumor cells and control cells as probes for fluorescence in situ hybridization on DNA chips loaded with thousands of defined DNA fragments. Comparison of the fluorescence intensities of both probes enables researchers to detect DNA losses and gains in tumor cells.

In 2004, **Dr. Frank Lyko** was lauded by the U.S. magazine "Technology Review" as one of the 100 top young innovators of the world. In the U.S., this is one of most prestigious distinctions for young scientists. For his discovery of the DNA methylation system in *Drosophila*, he was awarded the 2003 **Karl**

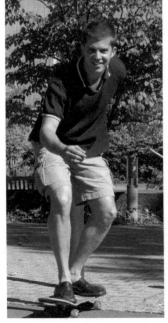

Freudenberg Prize, worth 6,000 euros, by the Heidelberg Academy of Sciences. One year earlier he had received the EUR 16,000 **Heinz Maier Leibnitz Prize** by the Deutsche Forschungsgemeinschaft. Frank Lyko's research work is focused on methyltransferases, whose activity controls the regulation of numerous genes. In tumor cells, in particular, genes that play a critical role for controlling cell growth are switched off by overactive methyltransferases.

Professor Otmar D. Wiestler, Scientific Director of the German Cancer Research Center, was awarded the translational part of the **2004 German Cancer Award** for his contributions to quality assurance in brain tumor diagnosis. Wiestler established the Brain Tumor Reference Center in Bonn, which has helped to enhance the quality and reliability of neuropathological diagnostics. The quality of therapy studies su-

pervised by the Center also benefits from these advances.

2003

Professor Hans-Peter Meinzer, head of the Division of Medical and Biological Informatics, jointly with his coworkers, **Matthias Thorn**, **Max Schöbinger** and **Tobias Heimann**, was awarded the **doIT Software Award** worth 15,000 euros. The prize, awarded by the Competence Center for Media, IT and High Tech of the State of Baden-Wuerttemberg, recognizes the development of the "OrgaNicer" software for liver surgery plan-

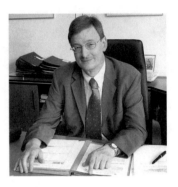

Bottom, from left to right:
Tobias Heimann, Dr. Matthias Thorn,
Prof. Hans-Peter Meinzer,
Max Schöbinger

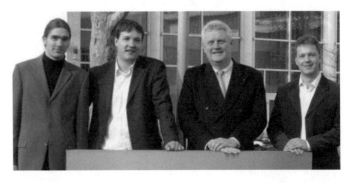

ning. From slice images of each individual patient, the program produces individual, three-dimensional views of the liver vessel system, which can be turned in any direction. This model facilitates spatial orientation for the surgeon before and during surgery.

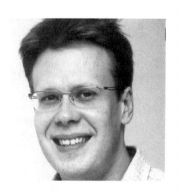

Dr. Daniel Gerlich, formerly of the Division of Theoretical Bioinformatics, was awarded the 2002 **Walther and Christine Richtzenhain Dissertation Prize** for his research on the dynamical organization of chromosomes in the nucleus. Gerlich shares the prize with **Dr. Axel Szabowski** (foto left), Division of Signal Transduction and Growth Control, who was honored for his work on gene regulation in skin cells.

Dr. Mathias Wind, Central Spectroscopy, was awarded the **Wolfgang Paul Study Award** of the German Association for Mass Spectrometry for his PhD thesis on the analysis of protein phosphorylation by means of mass spectroscopy.

Professor Lothar Schad, Division of Medical Physics in Radiation Oncology, received the 2003 Helmholtz Award, jointly with colleagues of Wuerzburg University. The prize, which consists of 15,000 euros, is awarded by the Helmholtz Fund e.V. and the Donors' Association for the Promotion of Sciences and Humanities in Germany. It was awarded for the development of a technology that facilitates qualitative and quantitative determination of a patient's coronary blood flow and, thus, detection of functional defects of the coronary vessels.

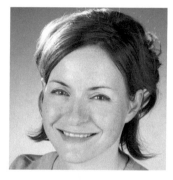

Dr. Selma Ugurel, Clincal Cooperation Unit "Dermato-Oncology", was awarded the **Research Award of the Fondation LaRoche-Posay**, which consists of a EUR 8,000 cash gift, for her studies on factors determining the course of malignant melanoma.

The German Association for Mass Spectrometry honored **Professor Wolf-Dieter Lehmann**, Central Spectroscopy, with the **Applied Biosystems Life Science Award** 2003. Lehman received the prize worth 5,000 euros for his application of mass spectrometry in the biosciences.

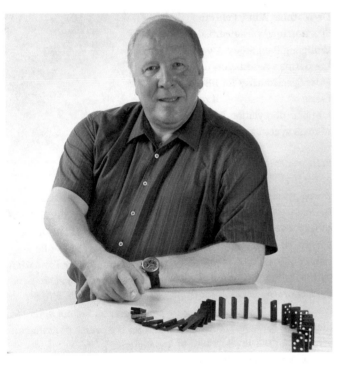

Professor Christof Niehrs, head of the Division of Molecular Embryology, was awarded the 2003 **Gottfried Wilhelm Leibniz Award** for his research work in the area of developmental biology. With an award amount of 1.55 million euros, this prize of the Deutsche Forschungsge-

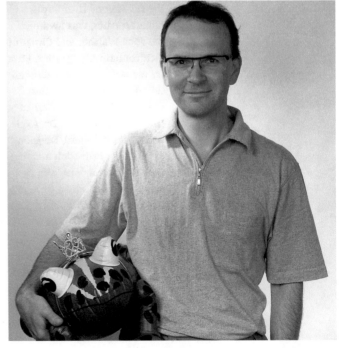

The EUR 250 000 **Lautenschlaeger Research Award Forschungspreis** 2003 was awarded to **Professor Peter Krammer**, head of the Division "Immunogenetics". Krammer was honored for his breakthroughs in research on apoptosis, or programmed cell death (see box on page 94).

Manfred Lautenschlaeger, founder of MLP, a financial services company, has intended the valuable prize for internationally recognized scientists of Heidelberg University and renowned researchers from other countries, who are connected to Heidelberg University through scientific collaborations.

meinschaft is the most valuable research award in Germany.

Using the clawed frog *Xenopus* as a model, Christof Niehrs is studying genes that play a role in embryonic development of vertebrates. To this end, he first developed a gene expression screening method which enabled him to identify developmental control genes in a semi-automated manner. Thus, he discovered, among others, the so-called 'Dickkopf' gene, which plays a role in the embryo's head formation. If 'Dickkopf' (which is the German word for 'thick head') is artificially activated, this leads to the formation of enlarged heads in the tadpoles. 'Dickkopf' is presumed to play a corresponding role in humans, since the vertebrate blueprints are very much alike. 'Dickkopf' is part of the wnt signaling cascade, which also plays a role in tumor development. For this work, Christof Niehrs had already received the Research Award of the State of Baden-Wuerttemberg in 2002.

PD Dr. Marco Essig, Radiology Division, was awarded the **Agfa Medical Imaging Grant** by the European Congress of Radiology. Marco Essig received the EUR 10 000 prize for his work in the area of contrast-enhanced dynamic MR angiography for vessel malformations of the brain.

The Deutsche Krebsgesellschaft honored **Professor Wolfgang Schlegel**, head of the Division of Medical Physics in Radiation Oncology, with the clinical part of the 2003 **German Cancer Award**. The prize, worth 7,500 euros, is awarded to Schlegel to recognize his achievements in

the enhancement of precision radiotherapy (see box on page 119).

2002

Dr. Uwe Engelmann (foto bottom), **André Schröter** and **Tilmann Schweitzer** were awarded the 2002 European IST Prize worth 5,000 euros for the development of Mobile-CHILI, a data transmission system for radiologists. Mobile-CHILI facilitates wireless transmission of medical images from the hospital to a mobile calculator sized device, enabling radiologists to receive and analyze images while traveling.

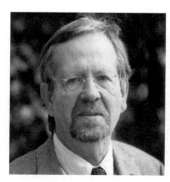
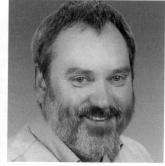

The German Cancer Research Center – Facts and Figures

Staff *as of Dec. 31, 2005*

Total Staff _____ 1830

Staff scientists without
doctoral students _____ 553

Doctoral students _____ 264

Scientific infrastructure __ 545

Management support ____ 140

Technical and
central services _____ 119

Apprentices _____ 126

Diploma students _____ 83

In 2005, there were **131 visiting
scientists** from **43 nations**
working at the DKFZ.

Collaborations with Industry

Since 1983, **11 companies**
have been founded as spin-
offs from the Center. They
provide about **150 jobs** today.

Technology Transfer

The DKFZ has filed about
**1050 German and foreign
patents** and has concluded
88 license agreements.

Funding 2005

Program-based funding
*Federal Government: 90%, State of
Baden-Wuerttemberg: 10%*
95.3 million Euro

Project funding (External funds)
*Federal or State governments, DFG,
EU, German Cancer Aid, etc.*
21.3 million Euro

Own revenues
*License revenues, patient care,
donations and bequests*
9.0 million Euro

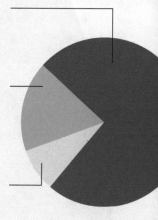

Expenditure 2005

Personnel expenses 72.8 million Euro

Material expenses 42.1 million Euro

Investment goods 10.7 million Euro

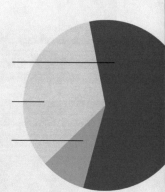

ISBN: 3-7985-1643-X

Published by:
Deutsches Krebsforschungszentrum
Im Neuenheimer Feld 280
D-69120 Heidelberg
presse@dkfz.de
www.dkfz.de

Editorial responsibility:
Dr. Julia Rautenstrauch,
Head of Press and Public Relations

Concept:
Dr. Sibylle Kohlstädt

Editors:
Dr. Sibylle Kohlstädt
Elisabeth Hohensee

Photo Editing:
Dagmar Anders

Authors:
Dagmar Anders
Dr. Birgit Hiller
Dr. Sibylle Kohlstädt
Dr. Stefanie Reinberger

Translation:
Stefanie v. Kalckreuth
Angela Lahee, PhD
special thanks to Margaret Vazansky

Layout Design:
UNIT Werbeagentur GmbH, Weinheim
www.unit-werbeagentur.de

Photos and Figures:
Yan de Andres, except
page 7, 13, 204 top right, 206: Brigitte Engelhardt;
page 8 to 10 and 14 to 17: Klaus Tschira Stiftung gGmbH/Stefan Kresin;
page 116 and 118: Markus Kirchgessner;
page 120 to 122: Clinical Cooperation Unit Radiation Oncology;
page 137: Division of Medical and Biological Informatics;
page 151, 154–158: Media Center of Heidelberg University Hospitals;
page 197 to 199: Philipp Rothe;
page 200 left: Uwe Dettmar;
page 200 center: Josef Wiegand;
page 202, 204 bottom right, 205, 207 right: private

© Deutsches Krebsforschungszentrum, Heidelberg 2006

Printed by: abcdruck GmbH, Heidelberg

Printed in the United States
by Baker & Taylor Publisher Services